AF181912

GROWTH DISORDERS AND ACROMEGALY

Edited by **Ahmed R.G.** and **Ahmet Uçar**

Growth Disorders and Acromegaly
http://dx.doi.org/10.5772/intechopen.78180
Edited by Ahmed R.G. and Ahmet Uçar

Contributors

Jesús Devesa, Belinda M. Contreras-Garza, Hugo Alberto Barrera-Saldaña, Silvia A. Barrera Barrera, Maria Dolores Gómez Roig, Edurne Mazarico, Mayank Choubey, Claire Briet, Valentine Suteau, Patrice Rodien, Yutaka Takahashi, Masaaki Yamamoto, Edward Laws, John Kilgallon, Ahmed R.G.

© The Editor(s) and the Author(s) 2020
The rights of the editor(s) and the author(s) have been asserted in accordance with the Copyright, Designs and Patents Act 1988. All rights to the book as a whole are reserved by INTECHOPEN LIMITED. The book as a whole (compilation) cannot be reproduced, distributed or used for commercial or non-commercial purposes without INTECHOPEN LIMITED's written permission. Enquiries concerning the use of the book should be directed to INTECHOPEN LIMITED rights and permissions department (permissions@intechopen.com).
Violations are liable to prosecution under the governing Copyright Law.

(cc) BY

Individual chapters of this publication are distributed under the terms of the Creative Commons Attribution 3.0 Unported License which permits commercial use, distribution and reproduction of the individual chapters, provided the original author(s) and source publication are appropriately acknowledged. If so indicated, certain images may not be included under the Creative Commons license. In such cases users will need to obtain permission from the license holder to reproduce the material. More details and guidelines concerning content reuse and adaptation can be found at http://www.intechopen.com/copyright-policy.html.

Notice

Statements and opinions expressed in the chapters are these of the individual contributors and not necessarily those of the editors or publisher. No responsibility is accepted for the accuracy of information contained in the published chapters. The publisher assumes no responsibility for any damage or injury to persons or property arising out of the use of any materials, instructions, methods or ideas contained in the book.

First published in London, United Kingdom, 2020 by IntechOpen
IntechOpen is the global imprint of INTECHOPEN LIMITED, registered in England and Wales, registration number: 11086078, 7th floor, 10 Lower Thames Street, London,
EC3R 6AF, United Kingdom
Printed in Croatia

British Library Cataloguing-in-Publication Data
A catalogue record for this book is available from the British Library

Additional hard and PDF copies can be obtained from orders@intechopen.com

Growth Disorders and Acromegaly, Edited by Ahmed R.G. and Ahmet Uçar
p. cm.
Print ISBN 978-1-83880-583-8
Online ISBN 978-1-83880-584-5
eBook (PDF) ISBN 978-1-83880-585-2

We are IntechOpen, the world's leading publisher of Open Access books

Built by scientists, for scientists

4,800+
Open access books available

122,000+
International authors and editors

135M+
Downloads

151
Countries delivered to

Our authors are among the
Top 1%
most cited scientists

12.2%
Contributors from top 500 universities

CLARIVATE ANALYTICS
BOOK CITATION INDEX
INDEXED

WEB OF SCIENCE™

Selection of our books indexed in the Book Citation Index
in Web of Science™ Core Collection (BKCI)

Interested in publishing with us?
Contact book.department@intechopen.com

Numbers displayed above are based on latest data collected.
For more information visit www.intechopen.com

For EU product safety concerns:
IN TECH d.o.o., Prolaz Marije Krucifikse Kozulić 3, 51000 Rijeka, Croatia,
info@intechopen.com or visit our website at intechopen.com.

Meet the editors

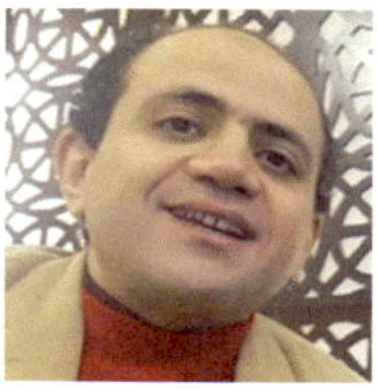

Prof. Dr Ahmed RG received his Ph.D. in Developmental Biology (Developmental-Toxicology/-Endocrinology) from Beni-Suef University, Egypt and received research training (postdoctoral fellowship) as a visiting scholar at the Katholic University, Belgium. Also, he has outstanding records of scientific and academic accomplishments with multiple research funding projects, numerous publications (books/papers) in highly prestigious journals, and various presentations in both national and international conferences. He is a member of several eminent societies, organizations, and schools. He has also served as a scientific editor and reviewer for national and international research institutions. He has been awarded several international prizes as follows:

2019-2020: Bentham Ambassador in Bentham Science Publishers.
2019: International Academic Mentor-Publons (Web of Science).
2018: Publons Peer Review Award (one of the top 1% of peer reviewers in assorted) [Honoring the Sentinels of Science and Research].
2018: Certified PUBLONS Academy Peer Reviewer.
2017: Publons Peer Review Award (one of the top 1% of peer reviewers in Science and Research) [Honoring the Sentinels of Science and Research].
2010: Honor from Society for Endocrinology, UK.

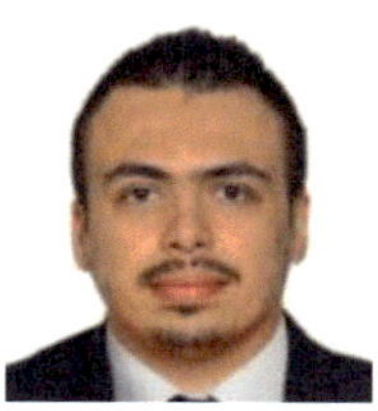

Prior to working at a major university of health sciences, Associate Prof. Ahmet Uçar received his degrees in pediatrics and then in pediatric endocrinology, achieving high honors at the national exams. He has been actively working in the field of pediatric endocrinology and diabetes, and he has contributed significantly to the definition of the characteristics of pubertal variants in children. He successfully completed a thesis on Turner syndrome, which has dramatically increased his interest in and dedication to Turner syndrome ever since. He is an active member of the Turner Syndrome Study Group in Turkey. He is also a member of the Endocrine Society and the European Society of Paediatric Endocrinology.

Contents

Preface

This book, *Growth Disorders and Acromegaly*, aims to provide an overview of the recent progress in growth disorders including growth hormone deficiency (GHD) and acromegaly, and worldwide research in growth failure, with a focus on different research areas relevant to these problems. These include the effects of growth hormone (GH) and its deficiency on the brain, cardiovascular system, female gonadal system (ovarian functioning), liver, kidney, adrenal gland, skeletal muscles, bones, hematopoietic system, and gastrointestinal system in children and adults. Also, this book reviews the causes and diagnoses of fetal growth defect including intrauterine growth restriction (IUGR) and fetal small for-gestational-age (SGA). It describes the role of the pituitary/placental human GH (hGH) and insulin-growth factor-1 (IGF-1) gene families during pregnancy. The authors have also contributed articles not only on the GH replacement therapy during pregnancy but also on the role of hGH locus in pioneering personalized medicine. This book proposes the impact of GH on germ cell proliferation/migration, testicular development, pubertal maturation, testicular steroidogenesis, and erectile function. It follows the impact of GH/Insulin/IGF-1 signaling in the regulation of testicular metabolic and energy status. Finally, this book illustrates the therapeutic potentials of GH on reproductive health and male infertility, the pegvisomant, colorectal neoplasms in acromegaly, epidemiology and underlying mechanisms and the surgical managements of acromegaly.

Ahmed, R.G.
Prof. Dr. of Developmental and Experimental Biology
Division of Anatomy and Embryology, Zoology department
Faculty of Science, Beni-Suef University, Egypt

Ahmet Uçar
MD, Associate Professor
University of Health Sciences, Şisli Hamidiye Etfal Education and Research Hospital
Pediatric Endocrinology and Diabetes Clinic, Istanbul, Turkey

Section 1

Introduction

Chapter 1

Introductory Chapter: Growth Disorders

Ahmed R.G.

Additional information is available at the end of the chapter

http://dx.doi.org/10.5772/intechopen.91661

For most of the last decade, the field of growth disorders has evolved with more decisive signs of its detrimental potential to the health and development of fetuses, neonates, childhoods, and adults. This introductory chapter is, briefly, embracing themes on the growth disorders including growth hormone deficiency (GHD) and fetal growth restriction (intrauterine growth restriction (IUGR)). It then goes on to cover the effects of GHD or IUGR on different biological systems.

1. Harmful effects of GHD

The numerous actions of GH and insulin-growth factor-1 (IGF-1) play an important role in the health and development of offspring/individual [1–7]. The disorder in this axis/GHD during the development caused several complications including weight defect and developmental distortion [8–12]. A systemic GHD can induce hypersensitivity (mechanical and thermal) during the early postnatal period [13]. Also, GHD can decrease the minerals in bones and increase the risk of fracture in adults [14]. The harmful actions of GHD are reinforced in the presence of hypopituitarism [14–16].

2. IUGR and GH treatment (GHT)

On the other hand, IUGR disrupted the neurodevelopment processes (proliferation, migration, and maturation) [17–20]. IUGR/GHD can cause fetal small for gestational age (SGA) [21] and increase the risk of cardiovascular, renal, visual, and mental diseases [22]; diabetes mellitus/obesity (increase in fat mass) [23, 24]; metabolic inflammation [25]; liver dysfunction [26]; mitochondrial imbalance (impair oxygen transport capacity) [27]; or immune problems [28, 29]. Moreover, GHD can delay the development and maturation of the male reproductive system [30] and the female reproductive system [31, 32]. The GHT is more effective on the female fertility [31], sperm efficiency [33], and mood and cognitive behavior in patients with

IntechOpen

© 2020 The Author(s). Licensee IntechOpen. This chapter is distributed under the terms of the Creative Commons Attribution License (http://creativecommons.org/licenses/by/3.0), which permits unrestricted use, distribution, and reproduction in any medium, provided the original work is properly cited.

GHD [34]. The outcome results of GHT depend on the age, gender, body mass index (BMI), muscle/bone index, and waist circumference. However, studies of possible effects of GHT on the gonads (sperm/ova quality) and fetal growth patterns in pregnancy are scarce.

Thus, the current *Growth Disorders* book will be of consciousness to scientists, embryologists, neuroendocrinologists, neurotoxicologists, and physicians coveting to follow recent publications in this field. This book explores in more detail the effects of GH and its deficiency on the brain, cardiovascular system, female gonadal system (ovarian functioning), liver, kidney, adrenal gland, skeletal muscles, bones, hematopoietic system, and gastrointestinal system in children and adults. Also, this book reviews the causes and diagnoses of fetal growth defect including IUGR and SGA. It describes the role of the pituitary/placental human GH (hGH) and IGF-1 gene family during pregnancy. Another theme of interest in this book is related to the impact of GH on germ cell development (proliferation, migration, and maturation), testicular development, pubertal maturation, testicular steroidogenesis, and erectile function. It follows the role of GH/Insulin/IGF-1 axis in the testicular activity. Finally, this book will discuss the impact of GH replacement therapy during pregnancy and its therapeutic potentials on reproductive health and male infertility.

Author details

Ahmed R.G.

Address all correspondence to: ahmedragab08@gmail.com

Division of Anatomy and Embryology, Faculty of Science, Zoology Department, Beni-Suef University, Beni-Suef, Egypt

References

[1] Caicedo D, Díaz O, Devesa P, Devesa J. Growth hormone (GH) and cardiovascular system. International Journal of Molecular Sciences. 2018;**19**:pii. E290

[2] Devesa J, Almengló C, Devesa P. Multiple effects of growth hormone in the body: Is it really the hormone for growth? Clinical Medicine Insights: Endocrinology and Diabetes. 2016;**9**:47-71

[3] Laron Z, Galatzer A. Growth hormone, somatomedin and prolactin—Relationship to brain function. Brain & Development. 1985;**7**:559-567

[4] Lobie PE, Garcia-Aragon J, Lincoln DT, Barnard R, Wilcox JN, Waters MJ. Localization and ontogeny of growth hormone receptor gene expression in the central nervous system. Brain Research. Developmental Brain Research. 1993;**74**:225-233

[5] Mateus J, Newman RB, Zhang C, Pugh SJ, Grewal J, Kim S, et al. Fetal growth patterns in pregnancy-associated hypertensive disorders: NICHD Fetal Growth Studies. American Journal of Obstetrics and Gynecology. 2019;**221**:635.e1-635.e16

[6] Neale J, Pais SMA, Nicholls D, Chapman S, Hudson LD. What are the effects of restrictive eating disorders on growth and puberty and are effects permanent? A systematic review and meta-analysis. Journal of Adolescent Health. 2020;**66**:144-156

[7] Savaheli S, Ahmadiani A. Obsessive-compulsive disorder and growth factors: A comparative review. Behavioural Brain Research. 2019;**372**:111967

[8] Ahmed RG, El-Gareib AW, Shaker HM. Gestational 3,3′,4,4′,5-pentachlorobiphenyl (PCB 126) exposure disrupts fetoplacental unit: Fetal thyroid-cytokines dysfunction. Life Sciences. 2018;**192**:213-220. DOI: 10.1016/j.lfs.2017.11.033

[9] Ahmed RG, El-Gareib AW. Gestational arsenic trioxide exposure acts as a developing neuroendocrine-disruptor by downregulating Nrf2/PPARγ and upregulating Caspase-3/NF-κB/Cox2/BAX/iNOS/ROS. Dose-Response. 2019;**17**(2):1559325819858266. DOI: 10.1177/1559325819858266

[10] Ahmed RG, El-Gareib AW. Maternal carbamazepine alters fetal neuroendocrine-cytokines axis. Toxicology. 2017;**382**:59-66. DOI: 10.1016/j.tox.2017.03.002

[11] Ahmed RG. Gestational caffeine exposure acts as a fetal thyroid-cytokine disruptor by activating caspase-3/BAX/ Bcl-2/Cox2/NF-κB at ED 20. Toxicology Research. 2019;**8**:196-205. DOI: 10.1039/c8tx00227d

[12] Ahmed RG. Overdoses of acetaminophen disrupt the thyroid-liver axis in neonatal rats. Endocrine, Metabolic & Immune Disorders Drug Targets. 2019;**19**(5):705-714. DOI: 10.2174/1871530319666190212165603

[13] Ford ZK, Dourson AJ, Liu X, Lu P, Green KJ, Hudgins RC, et al. Systemic growth hormone deficiency causes mechanical and thermal hypersensitivity during early postnatal development. IBRO Reports. 2019;**6**:111-121

[14] Tritos NA. Focus on growth hormone deficiency and bone in adults. Best Practice & Research Clinical Endocrinology & Metabolism. 2017;**31**:49-57

[15] Vestergaard P, Jorgensen JO, Hagen C, et al. Fracture risk is increased in patients with GH deficiency or untreated prolactinomasea case-control study. Clinical Endocrinology. 2002;**56**:159-167

[16] Wuster C, Abs R, Bengtsson BA, et al. The influence of growth hormone deficiency, growth hormone replacement therapy, and other aspects of hypopituitarism on fracture rate and bone mineral density. Journal of Bone and Mineral Research. 2001;**16**:398-405

[17] Dieni S, Rees S. Dendritic morphology is altered in hippocampal neurons following prenatal compromise. Journal of Neurobiology. 2003;**55**:41-52. DOI: 10.1002/neu.10194

[18] Lister JP, Blatt GJ, DeBassio WA, Kemper TL, Tonkiss J, Galler JR, et al. Effect of protein malnutrition on numbers of neurons in the principal layers of the adult rat hippocampal formation. Hippocampus. 2005;**15**:393-403. DOI: 10.1002/hipo.20065

[19] Mallard C, Loeliger M, Copolov D, Rees S. Reduced number of neurons in the hippocampus and the cerebellum in the postnatal guinea-pig following intrauterine growth-restriction. Neuroscience. 2000;**100**:327-333. DOI: 10.1016/S0306-4522(00)00271-2

[20] Sizonenko SV, Borradori-Tolsa C, Bauthay DM, Lodygensky G, Lazeyras F, Huppi P. Impact of intrauterine growth restriction and glucocorticoids on brain development: Insights using advanced magnetic resonance imaging. Molecular and Cellular Endocrinology. 2006;**254-255**:163-171. DOI: 10.1016/j.mce.2006.04.035

[21] de Bie HMA, Oostrom KJ, Delemarrre-van de Waal HA. Brain development, intelligence and cognitive outcome in children born small for gestational age. Hormone Research in Pædiatrics. 2010;**73**:6-14. DOI: 10.1159/000271911

[22] Noeker M. Neurocognitive development in children experiencing intrauterine growth retardation and born small for gestational age: Pathological, constitutional and therapeutic pathways. Hormone Research. 2005;**64**(Suppl. 3):83-88. DOI: 10.1159/000089322

[23] Beshyah SA, Freemantle C, Thomas E, et al. Abnormal body composition and reduced bone mass in growth hormone deficient hypopituitary adults. Clinical Endocrinology. 1995;**42**:179-189. DOI: 10.1111/j.1365-2265.1995.tb01860.x

[24] Møller N, Jørgensen JO. Effects of growth hormone on glucose, lipid, and protein metabolism in human subjects. Endocrine Reviews. 2009;**30**:152-177. DOI: 10.1210/er.2008-0027

[25] Höybye C, Faseh L, Himonakos C, Pielak T, Eugen-Olsen P. Serum soluble urokinase plasminogen activator receptor (suPAR) in adults with growth hormone deficiency. Endocrine Connections. 2019;**8**:772-779. DOI: 10.1530/EC-19-0159

[26] Nishizawa H, Iguchi G, Murawaki A, Fukuoka H, Hayashi Y, Kaji H, et al. Nonalcoholic fatty liver disease in adult hypopituitary patients with GH deficiency and the impact of GH replacement therapy. European Journal of Endocrinology. 2012;**167**:67-74. DOI: 10.1530/EJE-12-0252

[27] Zueger T, Loher H, Egger A, Boesch C, Christ E. Regulation of fuel metabolism during exercise in hypopituitarism with growth hormone-deficiency (GHD). Growth Hormone & IGF Research. 2016;**29**:39-44

[28] Sohmiya M, Kato Y. Effect of long-term administration of recombinant human growth hormone (rhGH) on plasma erythropoietin (EPO) and haemoglobin levels in anaemic patients with adult GH deficiency. Clinical Endocrinology. 2001;**55**:749-754. DOI: 10.1046/j.1365-2265.2001.01417.x

[29] Szalecki M, Malinowska A, Prokop-Piotrkowska M, Janas R. Interactions between the growth hormone and cytokines—A review. Advances in Medical Sciences. 2018;**63**:285-289

[30] Bartlett JM, Charlton HM, Robinson IC, Nieschlag E. Pubertal development and testicular function in the male growth hormone-deficient rat. The Journal of Endocrinology. 1990;**126**:193-201. DOI: 10.1677/joe.0.1260193

[31] Giampietro A, Milardi D, Bianchi A, Fusco A, Cimino V, Valle D, et al. The effect of treatment with growth hormone on fertility outcome in eugonadal women with growth hormone deficiency: Report of four cases and review of the literature. Fertility and Sterility. 2009;**91**:390.e7-390.e11. DOI: 10.1016/j.fertnstert.2008.09.065

[32] Spiliotis BE. Growth hormone insufficiency and its impact on ovarian function. Annals of the New York Academy of Sciences. 2003;**997**:77-84. DOI: 10.1196/annals.1290.009

[33] Ovesen PG, Jørgensen JO, Ingerslev J, Orskov H, Christiansen JS. Growth hormone treatment of men with reduced sperm quality. Ugeskrift for Laeger. 1998;**160**:176-180

[34] Butler T, Harvey P, Cardozo L, Zhu Y-S, Mosa A, Tanzi E, et al. Epilepsy, depression, and growth hormone. Epilepsy & Behavior. 2019;**94**:297-300. DOI: 10.1016/j.yebeh.2019.01.022

Section 2

Growth Disorders

Chapter 2

Growth Hormone Deficiency: Is It Just a Problem of Growth Impairment? Part I

Jesús Devesa

Additional information is available at the end of the chapter

http://dx.doi.org/10.5772/intechopen.88837

Abstract

The concept that the growth hormone (GH) is a merely metabolic pituitary hormone with effects on the longitudinal growth of the organism until the end of puberty has been questioned in recent years. We know today that the expression of GH also occurs in virtually all organs and tissues where it performs very important autocrine/paracrine and even intracrine functions. GH acts on all organs and tissues, being particularly important in the development of the brain during the fetal period. In addition, the hormone, after interacting with its membrane receptor, is internalized together with its receptor, allowing it to reach the cell nucleus where it acts as a transcription factor. In the first part of this review, we will analyze the effects of GH on the brain, the cardiovascular system, and the gonadal system, as well as the adverse effects that occur in the GH deficiency not treated in children and adults. GH is absolutely necessary for a normal brain development and also for repairing the nervous system after an injury. Moreover, GH plays a very important role in the cardiovascular system, as well as in normal gonadal functioning.

Keywords: GH deficiency, IGF-I, GH and nervous system, GH and cardiovascular system, GH and gonadal functioning

1. Introduction

Almost a century ago it was reported that the treatment of rats with bovine anterior pituitary gland extracts led to an increase in the growth of the animals treated with these extracts [1]; however, it was not until 35 years later, when from these pituitary extracts, from humans, in this case, the factor responsible for this effect on growth could be isolated and administered to human dwarfs that then began to grow normally [2], but this growth factor had to be obtained

IntechOpen

© 2019 The Author(s). Licensee IntechOpen. This chapter is distributed under the terms of the Creative Commons Attribution License (http://creativecommons.org/licenses/by/3.0), which permits unrestricted use, distribution, and reproduction in any medium, provided the original work is properly cited.

from human cadavers, and it was not pure and safe for its therapeutic use, until in 1971 its primary sequence was characterized and became known as growth hormone (GH). After that, and due to the development of genetic engineering, it was possible to start producing, since 1981, using recombinant DNA technology, unlimited amounts of the pure and safe hormone, obtained both from prokaryotes and eukaryotes, to be used in the treatment of children with GH deficiency (GHD).

Soon, the clinical use of GH and preclinical investigations allowed to know that the hormone was not only responsible for the longitudinal growth of the organism, but also it is a metabolic hormone with a counterregulatory function (it produces hyperglycemia since it antagonizes the actions of insulin on tissue uptake of glucose and induces lipolysis and protein anabolism). Moreover, GH induces the expression of many different growth factors (such as insulin-like growth factor I [IGF-I]) and exerts direct effects on cellular proliferation, differentiation, and survival [3].

In the last years, several investigations modified this classical description of GH as the hormone responsible for growth. While there are no doubts about the fact that GHD children grow defectively until they are treated with GH, many data indicate that the GH-growing effect mainly depends on the GH-induced liver production of IGF-I. In turn, the liver production of IGF-I is conditioned by the nutritional status of the organism, particularly the hepatic metabolism of glucose, and IGF-I is the hormone responsible for the longitudinal growth of the organism, a fact clearly seen in children of short stature in whom a defect in the hepatic receptor for GH (GHR) impedes that GH induces hepatic IGF-I expression [4, 5]. In this situation there are high levels of plasma GH but extremely low levels of plasma IGF-I, a condition that also can be seen GHR null mice [6, 7]. The administration of recombinant IGF-I reverts this growth problem, as it happens in children with Laron syndrome. Moreover, growth velocity in obese children is normal, despite that obesity leads to decreased or practically absent GH secretion, but in them, plasma IGF-I level is high [8, 9]. On the contrary, undernourished children or anorexia nervosa patients present high GH secretion but extremely reduced plasma IGF-I levels leading to decreased growth velocity [10, 11]. Curiously, there have been reported cases in which growth is normal and the final height is even above the target height in patients with persistent untreated GHD and undetectable IGF-I levels [12]; these patients suffered combined pituitary hormone deficiencies after resection of craniopharyngiomas and hypothalamic tumors. This led the authors to suggest that growth factors different to GH, IGF-I, insulin, or prolactin could play a growth-promoting role [12].

Currently, there are some other important concepts that go further to the classical description of GH. For instance, we know that there is a peripheral expression of the hormone, in practically all the tissues and organs where it plays an autocrine/paracrine role in the cells [3]. Therefore, besides the pituitary GH, there is a peripheral GH system owning specific properties. On the other side, the hormone, after interacting with its GHR in the cell membrane, is internalized together with its receptor via the endosomal pathway [13–15]. Once inside the cell, the hormone, which has arrived from the plasma, and its GHR are translocated to the nucleus where they act as transcription factors [13]. Therefore, the detection of the GHR in a

http://dx.doi.org/10.5772/intechopen.88837

cell nucleus indicates that there has been a previous interaction between GH and its receptor at the level of the membrane of this cell. This concept is schematized in **Figure 1**.

Data from our group indicate, at least in rats, that once internalized, GH can undergo a tissue-specific proteolytic processing, which originates different molecular forms. The actions of these GH-derived forms are unknown, but the type of them depends on the sex and age of the animal [16].

A review of the multiple actions that GH performs in the organism, far beyond its classically defined effects, can be seen in [3, 17].

Of course, any child with GH deficiency should receive hormone replacement therapy, but this does not always happen, and in the case of adults whether or not they are GHD, GH secretion decreases gradually with age, after age 20 [18], which may have a causal relationship with cardiovascular events and neurodegenerative diseases typical of aging.

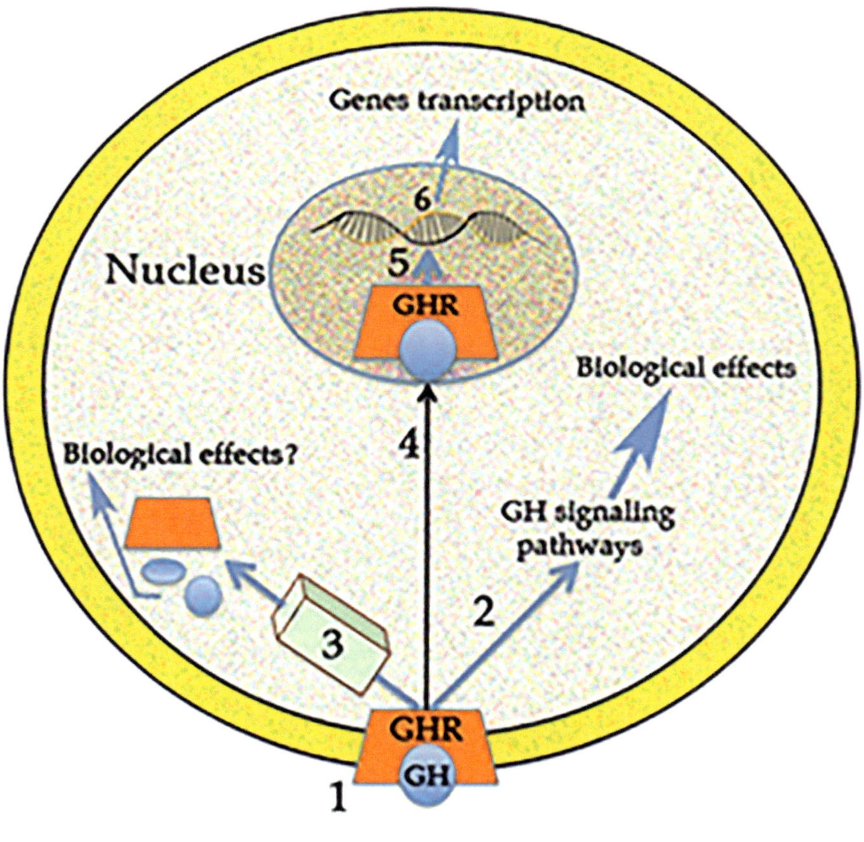

Figure 1. GH induces the translocation of its receptor to the nucleus of the cell. (1) After the binding of extracellular GH to its membrane receptor, a number of signaling pathways are activated (2) producing different biological effects. (3) GH and its receptor also are internalized via endosomes. There they suffer proteolytic degradations giving origin to shorter molecular forms which perhaps have a biological significance. (4) The internalization of GH and its receptor allows that they are translocated to the nucleus of the cell, where they act as transcription factors.

In this review we will analyze the possible harmful effects that the lack of GH can produce on a series of tissues and organs in the human body, without considering the known affectation of the longitudinal growth that occurs before puberty ends in untreated GHD children.

2. Untreated GH deficiency

Since many years ago, to establish that there is GHD implies the analysis of the amplitude of the GH response to at least two provocative stimuli, such as insulin-induced hypoglycemia, oral clonidine administration, propranolol plus exercise, etc. However, in many cases these tests produce a number of false-positive or false-negative responses [19]. This is due to the existence of an intrinsic hypothalamic-somatotroph rhythm, as we demonstrated in 1989 [20], that can condition the GH response to a provocative stimulus. As far as we know, the unique test in which no errors occur is the clonidine-GHRH test [21], but GHRH is no longer available in Spain and many other countries. The consequence of the lack of provocative tests that do not give uncertain results is that many children do not receive GH replacement therapy when in fact they need it.

2.1. GHD and nervous system functioning

Both GH and IGF-I play key roles in the development, maturation, and function of the brain [22, 23]. In fact, the presence of GHR in the brain is detected very early during neural development [24]. This implies that GH has to be present in the brain for interacting with its receptor [24]. This cerebral GH can come from the fetal anterior pituitary gland since the presence of this hormone in this gland has been identified toward week 7 postconception, and in plasma it is already detectable by 10 weeks of pregnancy [25, 26]. However, although it is well known that plasma GH can easily reach the central nervous system (CNS) [24], since GH-binding sites exist in the choroid plexus where they may act as carriers for plasma GH, a number of data indicate that the own GH is also synthesized in the CNS [27, 28], where, curiously, its regulation seems to be different to that of the pituitary GH. IGF-I is also synthesized in the CNS [29], and its expression, induced by GH, has been detected in neural stem cells from fetal human forebrains [30]. Both GH and IGF-I play a very important reparative role after a brain injury, a hypothesis postulated a long time ago [31] and later proved by many preclinical and clinical studies, regardless of whether the experimental animals or human patients were GHD or not [32–49].

Of interest here and before analyzing the effects of the lack of GH on the functioning of the brain is the case of children born small for gestational age (SGA) because of intrauterine growth retardation (IUGR) [50]. Together with several affectations that may occur later in their life (increased cardiovascular risk, diabetes mellitus type 2, and renal diseases), these children usually show decreased intelligence and cognition [51], especially manifested by the decrease of short-term memory. Animal studies in which IUGR had been induced showed that there was a decreased volume of both hippocampus and cerebellum [52, 53], a delayed neuronal migration to the cortex [54], and delayed dendritic and axonal outgrowth [53, 55, 56]; in addition, there was cortical thickness, decreased number of neurons [52, 53, 57, 58], and clearly reduced myelination [53, 55, 59, 60]. Similar results have been found in premature children with IUGR in whom there is a reduction of total brain volume, mainly in cerebral cortical gray matter [61–63], later traduced in attentional deficit, among other cerebral deficits, such as visual affectations. These concepts are schematized in **Figure 2**.

While it is now clear that the system GH/IGF-I plays a key role in the development of the fetal brain, although the pituitary GH does not exert any effect on the longitudinal growth of the fetus [3], there are no data indicating that IUGR children suffer from a deficient or absent GH production by the neural stem cells during the fetal development. It is also not known how the regulation of the cerebral production of this hormone takes place, but in any case and based on the data presented, it is reasonable to think that in these children with IUGR, a treatment with GH should be administered shortly after birth, to avoid and/or reduce the described deficits, something that generally does not occur. If a child with short stature is treated with GH, to increase his height, treatment usually does not begin before 4–5 years of age, but at these ages, the brain has already developed.

Similar brain deficiencies, although perhaps more marked, occur in untreated GHD children. Lack of attention and perception, deficient executive functions, and poor short-term memory are usual cognitive impairments observed in these children, who also show behavioral disorders. The same happens in GHD adults, in whom, in addition, there is a deteriorated psychological well-being. These impairments in cognitive functioning, especially subnormal memory speed, have been visualized by functional magnetic resonance imaging [64]. GH

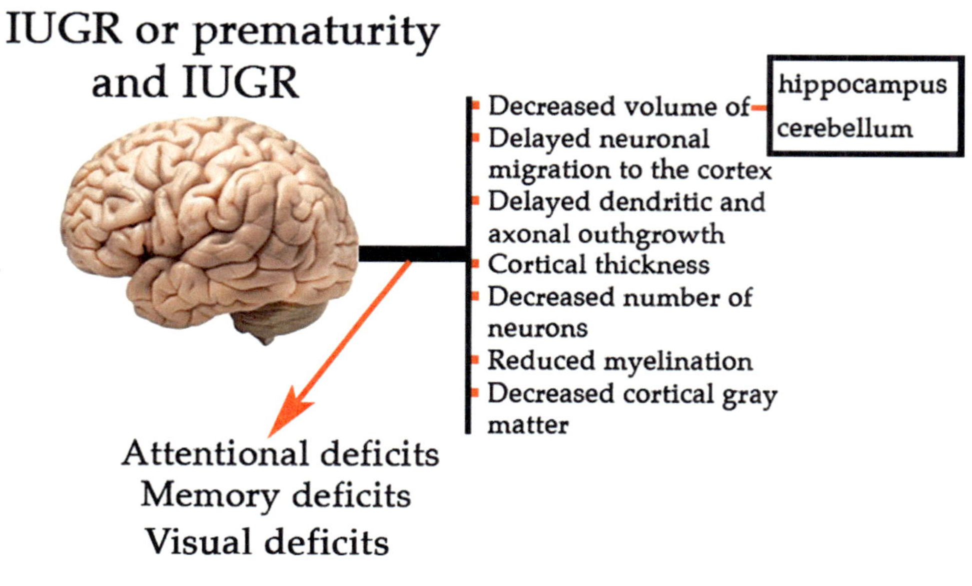

Figure 2. Schematic description of the affectations that may happen in children with IUGR or prematurity plus IUGR. Red arrow indicates the main alterations that may appear in these children.

replacement therapy recovers these deficits, both in children and adults, leading to marked improvements in the quality of life [65–71].

The question that should be asked now would be: how does GH exert these important actions in cognitive functions?

GH seems to be a very important regulator of hippocampus-dependent spatial learning and memory, therefore being able to revert memory deficiencies produced by alterations in cholinergic neurons and an imbalance in hippocampal glutamatergic and GABAergic synapses [72]; in addition, GH increases the blood flow to the brain and induces, via activation of PI3K/Akt pathways, the translocation of Glut4 vesicles to the plasma membrane for allowing the entry of glucose in neurons [73], and enhancement of excitatory synaptic transmission through NMDA receptors [74–77]. Although these studies have been carried out in rats, our recent data in an older woman support these effects of GH, not only in the hippocampus but also in practically all cortical areas, as measured by PET scans performed before GH administration and 1 month later [49]. It is likely that these effects of GH on cognition and the metabolic activity of the brain are also due to the effects of the hormone on the adult neurogenesis, both in physiological conditions and after a brain injury. It is also possible that, apart from the direct effects of GH in the brain, some of its actions are mediated by the induction of the expression of several neurotrophic factors, such as IGF-I, brain-derived neurotrophic factor (BDNF), erythropoietin (EPO), vascular endothelial growth factor (VEGF), epidermal growth factor (EGF), and some cytokines [3]. GH also modifies the levels of the main neurotransmitters (serotonin, noradrenaline, dopamine, the glutamatergic system, the opioid system, and the cholinergic system) in several brain areas, although the type of modification differs according to the brain area (for review, see [3]).

As stated above, the pituitary secretion of GH decreases progressively throughout aging; consequently, human adults suffer affectations in their cognitive functions, mainly short-term memory and their quality of life. Therefore, older people suffer a kind of GHD which can be reversed with GH replacement therapy.

There are other pathological situations in which a non-classic GHD appears, susceptible of being corrected, total or partially, with GH administration. This is the case, for instance, of children with cerebral palsy, traumatic brain injuries, stroke, spinal cord injuries above T5–T6, or neurosensorial hearing loss, and even injuries in central or peripheral nerves.

Data from our group indicate that in a large number of children with cerebral palsy, 70% of them lacked normal GH secretion [78]. We do not know if this GHD is a consequence of the neonatal injury or if it occurs as a result of the high spasticity that leads to a deficient production of IGF-I, but in any case GH administration in these children is very useful and helps to the kinesitherapy and the recovery of lost brain functions [40, 79]. Similar recoveries, after GH administration and rehabilitation, have been seen in traumatic brain injuries [35–37, 39, 41–44, 47] and after a stroke, both in rats [48] and humans [80, 81]. **Figure 3** shows the recovery of a 52-year-old man who, 1 year previously, had suffered an ischemic infarction of the left middle cerebral artery, which led to aphasia and right hemiplegia. We treated him with GH and rehabilitation, and 18 months later he had fully recovered, without any sequel.

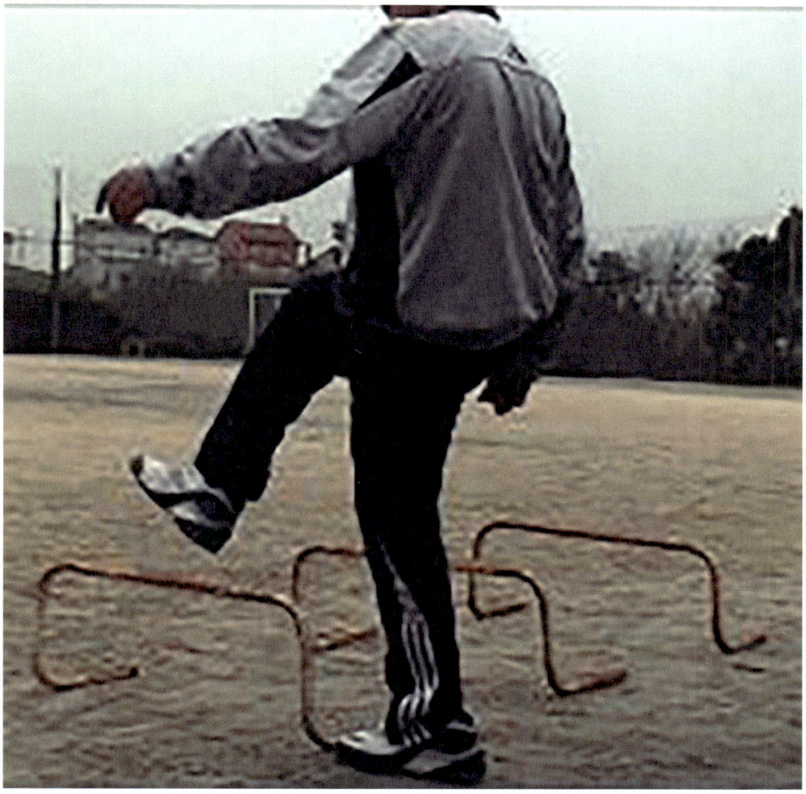

Figure 3. Recovery from an ischemic stroke. The patent suffered aphasia and right hemiplegia. He was treated with rehabilitation and GH (0.6 mg/day during 3 months, followed by 1 month without GH administration, and again another 3 months under GH treatment. This pattern was conducted over 18 months). At discharge he had recovered all lost functions. In the picture, it can be seen how the patient moves perfectly the right arm and leg, previously paralyzed.

In the case of the spinal cord, injuries above T5–T6, there is a loss of the afferent inputs from the spinal cord to the sympathetic ganglionic chain resulting in a decreased or absent supply of catecholamines to the hypothalamus. The result of this situation would be an increased hypothalamic somatostatin release and, consequently, deficient or insufficient GH secretion [82]. This GHD in patients with spinal cord injuries had been reported years ago [83, 84], but never were they treated with GH, until 2007, when we began to treat these patients with the hormone and rehabilitation, based on the fact that there are neural stem cells in the spinal cord ependyma whose proliferation and differentiation is stimulated by GH, with good or very good results in many cases (**Figure 4**), although we still have not published our results.

Recently, the administration of GH to this type of patients has been reported to be safe and effective [85]. The effects of GH on the spinal cord have been clearly demonstrated by our group in a young child affected by caudal regression syndrome at the L2 level [86]. The treatment started when the patient was 3 months old. Five years later and, even though the patient

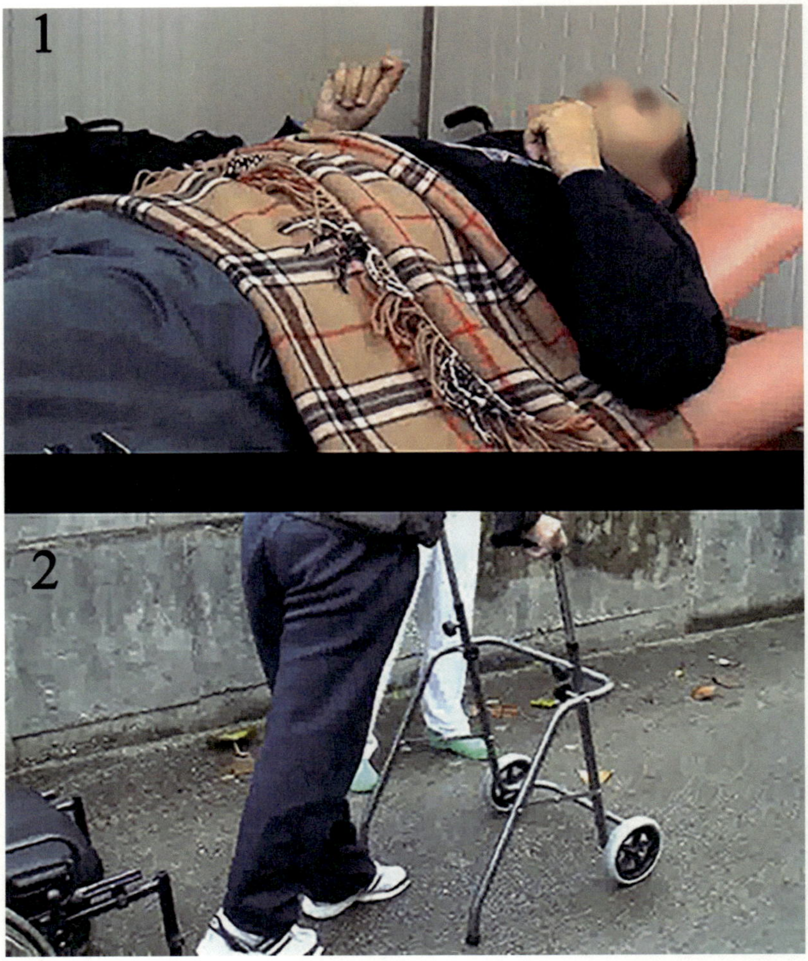

Figure 4. Recovery from a complete spinal cord injury (level C5–C6, ASIA A). The injury occurred 6 years before, at 16 years old. (1) The patient at admission. He could only move his arms but did not reach the mouth. He had a great spasticity. He was treated with rehabilitation and GH (1 mg/day, following the same pattern described in **Figure 3**). (2) Two years later he was able to walk with the help of a walker. Currently, 10 years after discharge, he walks 5 km/day, although he still needs the walker.

also suffered from a lack of sacral bone, he was able to walk with the help of a cane and to get up from the ground without help, has full sensitivity in the legs and feet, and has sphincter control. This indicates that, although the spinal column did not grow, new spinal roots were formed that fully innervated the legs, feet, and sphincters. These effects, the first case in the world, only can be attributed to GH.

Neurosensorial hearing loss is a quite common finding in children with perinatal problems and also in children with alterations in GH secretion or its signaling pathways [87, 88]. We treated with GH and specific auditory stimulation a child with cerebral palsy, beginning when he was 3.5 months old, and 14-months later he was fully normal [89]. Most likely hearing loss was recovered due to the effect of GH on the production of hair cells from stem cells existing in the cochlear sensory epithelium. These stem cells are present only in very young children and respond to GH proliferating and differentiating. This was the first known case in which hearing loss was recovered by the administration of this hormone.

GH is also a promising therapy for central and peripheral nerve injuries. For instance, a common finding in children with cerebral palsy is a delayed conduction from the retina to the occipital cortex, but we corrected it with the administration of GH and visual stimulation with a tachistoscope [90] (**Figure 5**).

In this case, it is likely that the hormone increased the number of fibers in the optical nerve and promoted myelination of them. A similar regeneration was obtained in an untreated GHD patient, 15 years after she suffered a brain surgery because of a bulbar astrocytoma (what was the cause of the GHD). The surgery produced paralysis of oropharyngeal structures, paralysis of vocal cords, and lack of primary esophageal peristalsis, because of iatrogenic

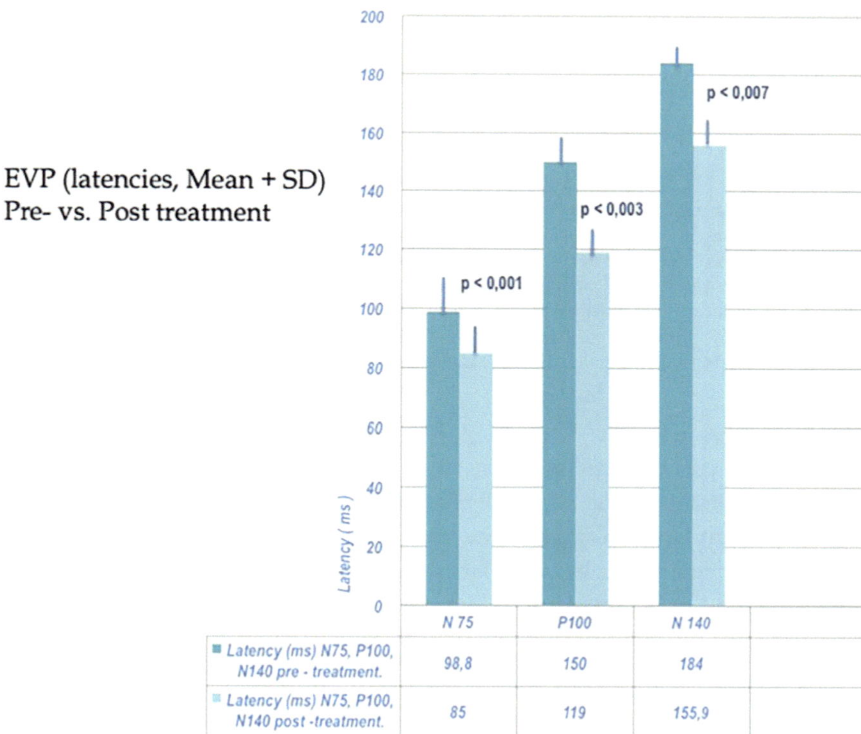

Figure 5. Evoked visual potentials (EVP) in 36 young children with cerebral palsy. Note the significant decrease in the conduction velocity from the retina to the occipital cortex, after being treated with GH (0.04 mg/kg/day) and visual stimulation with a tachistoscope. This indicates an increase in the number of fibers and myelination of the optical nerve.

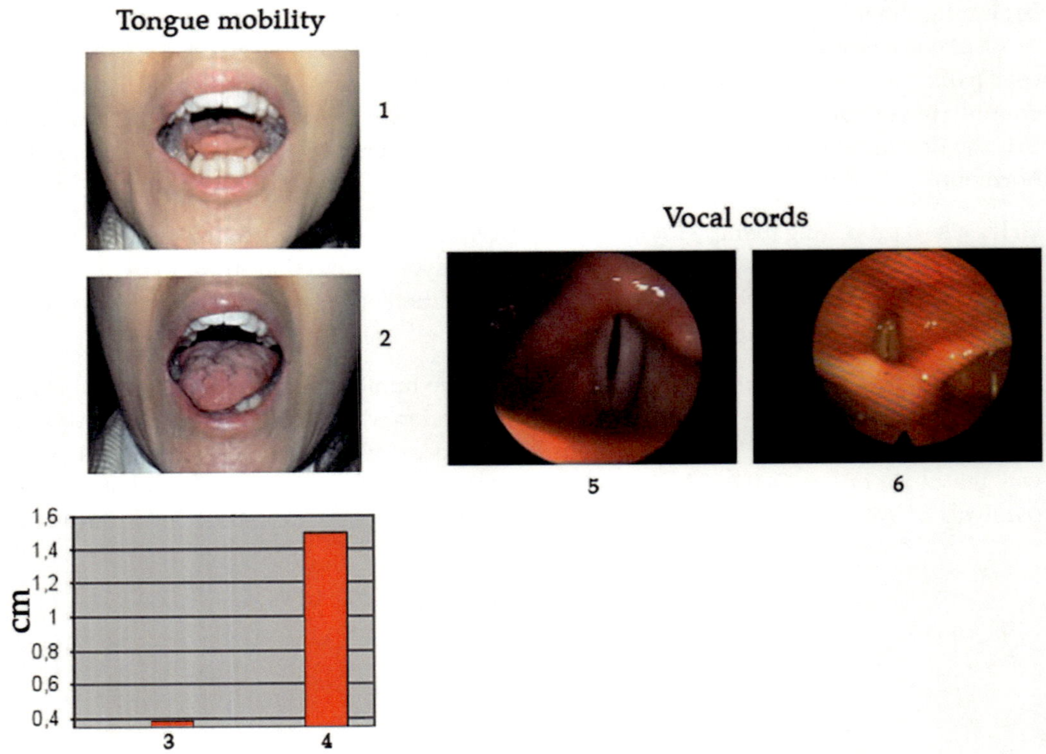

Figure 6. Recovery from cranial nerve pair damage 15 years after bulbar surgery. (1) The patient at admission was unable to move the tongue, it was atrophic, and the mouth continuously accumulated highly dense mucous saliva (sympathetic saliva). (2) Four months after being treated with GH (1 mg/day, 5 days/week) and speech therapy, the tongue had increased its size and showed important mobility; the patient began to speak and ceased to accumulate sympathetic saliva. (3) Indicates the inability to move the tongue forward (red rectangle). (4) Four months later these forward movements clearly improved (red rectangle). (5) At admission there was paralysis of the vocal cords. (6) Eight months later the vocal cords move normally. The patient was discharged practically recovered from her dysfunctions.

palsy of cranial nerve pairs IX, X, and XII. Therefore, the patient was unable to speak or swallow, her tongue was atrophic, and vocal cords were paralyzed. Moreover, her mouth was continuously full of sympathetic highly dense mucous saliva, and there was the need of nocturnal volumetric ventilation because of the severity and frequency of her sleep apneas. Eight months after beginning a treatment with GH and speech therapy, the patient was discharged practically recovered [91] (**Figure 6**).

Since the patient had undergone an intense oral rehabilitation for almost 15 years, without any success, it seems clear that the administration of GH was the factor responsible for the recovery of damaged cranial nerves.

We also demonstrated, in rats, that the administration of GH administration led to complete functional recovery of the sciatic nerves after their transection [92], promoting the appearance of a high number of axons and Schwann cells, while in the group of rats treated with placebo, a persistent paralysis of the affected limb was present.

In summary, from these and many other data, it is clear that GH is a hormone that plays many important roles in the development and functional maintenance of the nervous system, central and peripheral, and/or its repair when an injury exists. These effects have nothing to do with the longitudinal growth of the organism, but do not appear in untreated GHD children or adults when really they do need the replacement therapy with the hormone.

2.2. GHD and cardiovascular system

As it happens in the brain during fetal development, GH has direct effects in the heart of the fetus; the hormone induces myocardial growth and improves the cardiac function [93]. Fetal GH induces mRNA expression of specific contractile proteins, increases the force of cardiac contraction, and induces the phenoconversion of myosin toward the low ATPase activity V3 isoform [93]. This allows to increase the number of actin-myosin cross-bridges and their attachment time, enhances protein calcium sensitivity and calcium availability, and allows the myocardium to function at lower energy cost. Therefore, the fetal heart is able to beat at high frequency without spending too much energy. After birth, this changes, and myocardial remodeling occurs; the V1 myosin is then expressed, which implies a higher ATPase activity. Some of these effects of GH on the fetal heart may be produced by GH-induced IGF-I expression in the heart. The GH-IGF-I axis may also regulate cardiac metabolism, by increasing amino acid uptake, protein synthesis, cardiomyocyte size, and myocardial-specific gene expression. In addition, GH-induced IGF-I reduces apoptosis of cardiomyocytes, thus preventing myocyte loss, and increases the collagen deposition rate in the heart [94–99].

Although many of the aforementioned studies come from preclinical research, the important role that GH plays at the myocardial level can be easily observed by analyzing what happens in untreated GHD children and adults. In them, there is cardiac atrophy with a significant reduction in the left ventricle mass, relative wall thickness, and cavity dimensions, in comparison with age-, sex-, and height-matched controls [100–104]. These patients also have a low ejection fraction, low cardiac output, and high peripheral vascular resistance [100, 102–105]. As is logical, physical exercise increases these alterations; consequently, the intensity of exercise and its duration are reduced in both GHD children and adults [106, 107]. However, adult-onset GHD does not produce a reduction in cardiac mass. GH replacement therapy in GHD adults exerts significant positive effects on cardiac abnormalities, as it has been shown in several trials. The left ventricular mass increases, cardiac performance improves, and diastolic filling and systolic function also improve, both in GHD children and adults when they receive a GH treatment [100–102, 104, 105, 108] (**Figure 7**).

Therefore, and given the positive effects of GH on the heart, it is likely that GH treatment may be useful in patients with heart failure, even if they are not GHD. Many recent studies support such a possibility, and the treatment with GH has been proposed and carried out with very good results in untreated GHD children and adults with heart failure and also in patients suffering this affectation even though they are not GHD [109–117], although there are studies suggesting that this GH therapy only provides positive results in GHD patients [118].

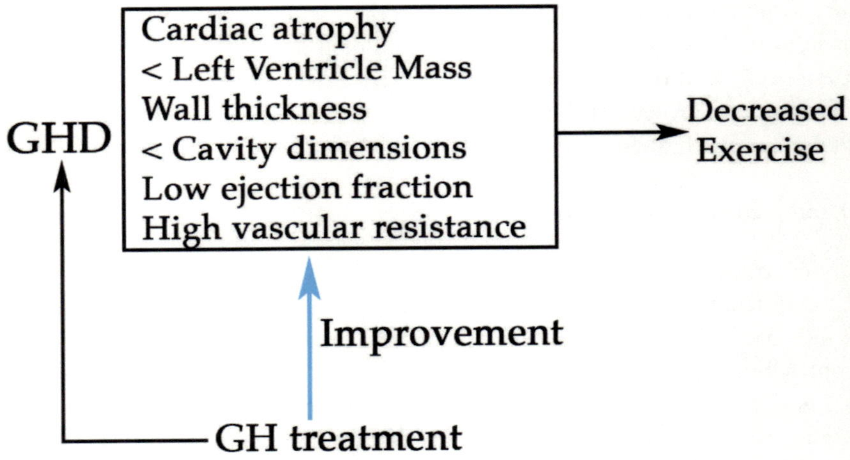

Figure 7. The effect of GH treatment on cardiovascular functioning in GHD patients. Untreated GHD patients suffer several important affectations in the heart. This leads to an increased cardiovascular risk and decreased exercise. GH administration reverts (blue arrow) these cardiac affectations and improves the quality of life in these GHD patients.

In any case, the interactions between the heart and GH are very complex. An example of it is the fact that the heart may condition body growth in children with heart diseases. This is due to the fact that, in these situations, cardiomyocytes produce and release a peptide known as GDF15, which inhibits liver signaling by GH; therefore, liver IGF-I is not released, and body growth is affected [119].

The GH/IGF-I system also exerts important actions at the vascular level. For instance, this system activates the production of nitric oxide (NO) that induces the relaxation of arterial smooth muscle cells; as a consequence, the vascular tone is reduced. In addition, NO inhibits the proliferation and migration of smooth muscle cells, decreases platelet adhesion, and decreases lipoxygenase activity and oxidized LDL cholesterol [120–124]. These are some of the reasons by which GHD patients show an abnormal vascular reactivity [125], although the lack of effect of GH on the expression of the vascular smooth muscle KATP channel may also be involved in this affected vascular tone observed in untreated GHD patients [126]. GHD have an increased risk of atherosclerosis and vascular mortality [127]. GH treatment restores the vascular resistance and vasodilation and even may reverse early atherosclerosis.

GHD patients present markedly increased muscle sympathetic nerve activity [128], which seems to be of central origin and perhaps is an important mechanism leading to secondary hypertension and increased cardiovascular morbidity in these patients. In fact, 1 year of treatment with GH induces, in adults GHD, an effect on decreasing sympathetic nerve activity in the muscular vascular bed [129].

GH also plays a significant role on angiogenesis, contributing to regulate vascular growth and function (for review, see [17]). Most likely this is the reason by which the skin of adult GHD patients shows reduced capillary density and permeability, and these are improved after treatment with GH [130]. Retinal vascularization is reduced in children and adults GHD [131, 132], although this may be a consequence of decreased IGF-I [132], since the vascular effects of GH may be exerted by other angiogenic agents induced by the hormone [17].

In summary, GH plays a very important role in the cardiovascular system, and untreated GHD patients suffer the consequences of the lack of the hormone and its mediators [109, 133, 134] and the risk of developing atherosclerosis, and suffering from cardiac affectations increases in them.

2.3. GHD and gonadal functioning

2.3.1. GHD and testicular functioning

In males, the effects of GH on testis seem to be different according to the species and the age of the individual. This is the case of rats and mice. Dwarf rats have small testis and normal spermatogenic function, suggesting that GH does not play a role in spermatogenesis during puberty and adult life, although the small testicular size may indicate that these animals have a small number of Sertoli cells, which in turn would indicate that GH may be important for the development of prepubertal testis [135]. However, homozygous GH-deficient mouse mutants (Snell dwarf mice) present infantile seminal vesicles, and spermatogenesis appears later in life [135]. From this study, the authors concluded that GHD only partially affects the reproductive axis, and this affectation occurs at an early age.

Unlike what happens in the CNS, plasma GH cannot easily access testicular cells within the blood-testis barrier. GH gene expression has been detected within the rat, human, and chicken testes [136, 137]. GHR has been detected in the human testis, mainly in Leydig cells [138]. Factors which regulate GH secretion are similarly expressed in the testis. This is the case of growth hormone releasing hormone (GHRH) found in the testis of rats, chicken, and humans [136, 137]. This testicular GHRH is capable of stimulating the pituitary release of GH, which indicates that it is similar or the same than the hypothalamic GHRH, but it is also able to induce the activity of adenylate cyclase (AC) in Sertoli cells [136]. At the testicular level, receptors for GHRH have been found in Leydig cells, Sertoli cells, germ cells, and even in the prostate, suggesting that this GHRH can exert specific actions on the testicle, different from those of GH itself [139]. Another inducer of pituitary secretion of GH, such as ghrelin, has also been found in mature Leydig cells of rat and human testis, where it has been shown that acting on its GHS-R type 1a receptor modulates the proliferation of Leydig cells and the expression of important testicular genes, such as the stem cell coding factor [140]. Interestingly, negative regulators of GH secretion and the actions of this hormone, such as somatostatin (SS) and its receptors (SSTR1–SSTR5), have been detected in Sertoli cells of mice [141]; treatment with somatostatin significantly promotes the apoptosis of these cells and decreases the expression of IGF-I together with a dose-dependent suppression of the mRNA level of the *kitl* gene, which is important in the regulation of spermatogenesis. These findings suggest that somatostatin and its receptors (mainly SSTR2 and SSTR5) play an important role in the regulation and development of Sertoli cells [141]. All these data indicate that practically all the components of the hypothalamus-somatotroph axis exist in the testicle, although it is

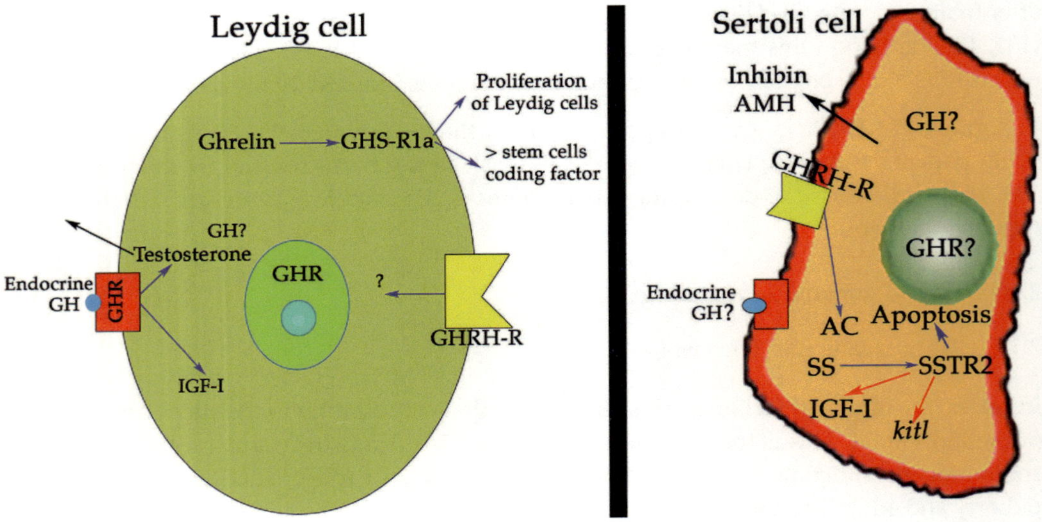

Figure 8. Hormonal factors involved in the functioning of testicular Leydig and Sertoli cells. Left: In Leydig cells there is expression of a number of hormones related to GH. There is GHR in the nucleus of these cells, indicating that there is GH expression in Leydig cells (GH?), although the nuclear GHR could proceed from the interaction of endocrine GH with its membrane receptor. This interaction leads to the expression of IGF-I inside the Leydig cell, and it is also responsible for the production of testosterone (induced by LH), which is secreted to the plasma. Interestingly, there are receptors for GHRH in the membrane of Leydig cells, although its role is unknown. In addition, another important inducer of GH secretion, such as ghrelin, has been found to be expressed in Leydig cells. Ghrelin acts (blue arrow) on its receptor GHS-R1a inducing the proliferation of Leydig cells and increasing the activation of stem cell coding factor. Right: As in Leydig cells there are GHR in the membrane of Sertoli cells; this may explain the presence of the GHR in the nucleus of these cells, although it is not well known, as it is not known if GH is expressed in Sertoli cells (GH?). In Sertoli cells there are receptors for GHRH (GHRH-R) which activate adenylate cyclase, although the effects produced are not known. Curiously, somatostatin (SS) and its receptors (mainly SSTR2 and SSTR5) are expressed in Sertoli cells. The interaction of SS with its receptors (blue arrow) leads to the inhibition of IGF-I and *kitl* gene expression (red arrows) and induces apoptosis of these Sertoli cells.

unknown exactly how they act and if there is any relationship with the similar endocrine axis. These concepts are shown in **Figure 8**.

Despite the fact that, in this regard, the testis seem to behave like a small hypothalamic-pituitary gland, endocrine GH promotes testicular growth and development and stimulates gametogenesis and steroidogenesis in the adult testis. These actions seem to be mediated by IGF-I, since it can recover testicular differentiation in fetal mice treated with GH antibodies and testicular growth in children with Laron syndrome [142, 143].

In vitro, GH is a potent steroidogenic factor that stimulates androgen and estradiol production by Leydig cells in a number of species including humans. In vivo, GH treatment has been seen to increase the production of testosterone, induced by chorionic gonadotropin, and seminal plasma volume, in fertile GHD human patients [144, 145]. Similar effects have been described in boys with GHD after being treated with GH [146]. However, and contrarily to what should be expected, GH treatment in hypopituitary or moderately obese men decreases the concentrations of total serum testosterone [147, 148]; most likely this effect is due to an increased aromatase activity and the resulting increased conversion of testosterone to estradiol [149]. In this study it was also found that high GH plasma levels were associated with reduced activity of the anti-Müllerian hormone (AMH), a marker of the Sertoli cells.

At this point it would be of interest to analyze if there is GH expression in the testis of GHD patients (children or adults) or experimental animals, both in cases of GHD due to a traumatic brain injury and a *GH* gene mutation or deletion, since it has been shown that in males born small for gestational age GH treatment does not affect the testicular production of inhibin and AMH [150]. That is, it seems that the pituitary GH does not play a key role in the testicular functioning, but acts as a co-gonadotropin that improves the secretion of gonadotropins (Gns), particularly LH, by acting directly or through IGF-I in the activation of GnRH pulse generator by means of the stimulation of hypothalamic kisspeptin [151].

It is also important to reflect that the GH variant GHV, seems to be the most abundant GH mRNA isoform in the human testis [152], while in chicken the GH 17 kDa variant is predominant [153].

In summary, from these data, it is likely that, in a normal man, endocrine GH synergizes with gonadotropins, potentiating the effects of these hormones on testicular cells, while the role of the testicular GH axis and its relationships with endocrine GH remain unknown.

2.3.2. GHD and ovarian functioning

The relationship between GH and ovarian functioning has been widely analyzed since many years ago. In humans, and in many other species, GH seems to play a direct role in the nuclear maturation of oocytes [154, 155]. In 1990, the existence of a strong immunoreactivity for the GH receptor at the nuclear level was described not only in rat oocytes but also in practically all the reproductive systems of the rats studied [156]. These data led to suggest that GH could play important and direct actions on reproduction. In human oocytes, the GHR has been detected in the membrane, in cumulus cells and in the nucleus in mature ovaries [157], confirming that GH has to act at this level improving nuclear maturation and the expansion of cumulus cells, as has been demonstrated in primates [158], and also improving the cytoplasmic maturation of mature oocytes [159]. There is a genetic expression of GHR in cumulus cells, mature oocytes, and preimplantation human embryos, in which the expression of GHR increases from the 4-day morula onwards [154]. This study led to the conclusion that, in humans, GH plays a role in the maturation of the oocyte and embryogenesis, from its early stages.

Most of the GH effects on the ovarian functioning are exerted by the hormone locally produced in the ovaries; however, plasma GH released by the pituitary gland or exogenously administered also plays an important role in the normal function of the female gonad and reproduction [160]. In fact, GH participates in the regulation of puberty and fertility, although these effects may depend on GH-induced changes in Gns secretion, directly or via IGF-I [161, 162].

Preclinical and clinical data indicate that an appropriate secretion of GH is needed for sexual maturation and maintenance of reproductive functions, while GH deficiency may affect the beginning of the puberty and can produce infertility. In humans, the interaction of GH-GHR in the ovary promotes the synthesis of sex steroids and induces gametogenesis, inhibits follicular apoptosis, and upregulates ovarian receptors for LH [160, 162, 163]. GHD women, in which puberty is delayed and the reproductive function is affected, recover a normal ovarian function when they are treated with GH [163]; the same happens in infertile eugonadal women with GH deficiency in whom GH treatment restores fertility and leads to successful pregnancies [164].

Although the onset of puberty in girls is a very complex process in which many factors participate (genetic, nutritional status, ethnicity, among others), there seems to be a relationship between increased GH secretion and puberty, since this hormone seems to act as a co-gonadotropin that enhances the effects of Gns on the ovarian production of sex steroids [165]. In fact, GH deficiency has been identified as the only cause of primary amenorrhea in three adolescent women in whom the secretion of gonadotropins was normal, suggesting that GH would play a complementary role to gonadotropins for the onset of menarche [166]. Therefore, and as stated above, GH deficiency negatively affects ovarian function in humans delaying sexual maturation and fertility, a situation that is reversed with GH replacement therapy. In addition, GH plays a very important role in ovarian angiogenesis, inducing the increased vascularization of one of the primary follicles that begin to maturate during a menstrual cycle allowing it to be the dominant follicle which will release the ovule (for review, see [167]).

GH also plays a role in the uterus, where the hormone acts very early in gestation. Both GH and GHR are expressed in the uterus, independently of the existence or not of pregnancy [3]. GH induces uterine hypertrophy facilitating the implantation of the embryo. In women with thin endometrium, the administration of GH leads to greater endometrium thickness; very early, the hormone leads to higher implantation rates and greater clinical pregnancy rates than with untreated patients [168]. These effects are due to the proliferation of endometrial cells and increased vascularization via induction of the expression of VEGF-A. The increased rates of implantation seem to be a consequence of GH-induced increased production of metalloproteinases and stimulation of trophoblast cells proliferation, thus allowing the formation of the blastocyst cavity and invasion of the endometrium, as it has been seen in mice [169].

In summary, GH plays very important roles in all stages of the ovarian development and functioning, and recent studies indicate that this hormone can be an important factor as adjuvant therapy for in vitro fertilization and embryo transfer in infertile women or poor ovarian responders. Untreated GHD females present delayed (or absent) onset of the puberty, and impaired fertility is more marked in female patients with childhood-onset hypopituitarism; they have lower fertility rates and less positive pregnancy outcomes [170]. GH replacement therapy reverts these alterations.

3. Conclusions

GH is a key hormone for the normal development of the brain and for repairing the nervous system when it suffers any injury. This hormone also contributes to the repair of the cardiovascular system, particularly increasing the blood flow by inducing the formation of collateral vessels that allow overcoming a circulatory obstruction and repairing the arterial intimate layer damaged by an arteriosclerotic process. In addition, the hormone plays an important role at the gonadal level in both sexes, perhaps more important in women, facilitating fertility. Untreated GHD patients suffer the consequences of the lack of the hormone when any of the organs here described is damaged, as it has been analyzed in this review.

Acknowledgements

We thank the therapists of Foltra Medical Center (Teo, Spain) and researchers from the Department of Physiology of the Faculty of Medicine of the University of Santiago de Compostela who contributed with their work to a large part of the information provided in this review. We also acknowledge the Foltra Foundation (Teo, Spain) for the help provided to write this review. This review has been funded by Foundation Foltra (Teo, Spain), grant F2019-7.

Conflict of interest

The author declares that there is no conflict of interest.

Author details

Jesús Devesa

Address all correspondence to: devesa.jesus@gmail.com

Scientific Direction, Medical Center Foltra, Teo, Spain

References

[1] Evans HM, Long JA. The effect of the anterior lobe administered intraperitoneally upon growth maturation, and oestrus cycles of the rat. The Anatomical Record. 1921;**21**:62-63

[2] Raben MS. Treatment of a pituitary dwarf with human growth hormone. The Journal of Clinical Endocrinology and Metabolism. 1958;**18**:901-903

[3] Devesa J, Almengló C, Devesa P. Multiple effects of growth hormone in the body: Is it really the hormone for growth? Clinical Medicine Insights: Endocrinology and Diabetes. 2016;**9**:47-71. DOI: 10.4137/CMED.S38201

[4] Laron Z, Pertzelan A, Mannheimer S. Genetic pituitary dwarfism with high serum concentration of growth hormone—A new inborn error of metabolism? Israel Journal of Medical Sciences. 1996;**2**:152-155

[5] Laron Z, Kauli R. Fifty seven years of follow-up of the Israeli cohort of Laron Syndrome patients—From discovery to treatment. Growth Hormone & IGF Research. 2016;**28**:53-56. DOI: 10.1016/jghir.2015.08.004

[6] Zhou Y, Xu BC, Maheshwari HG, He L, Reed M, Lozykowski M, et al. A mammalian model for Laron syndrome produced by targeted disruption of the mouse growth hormone receptor/binding protein gene (the Laron mouse). Proceedings of the National Academy of Sciences of the United States of America. 1997;**94**:13215-13220. DOI: 10.1073/pnas.94.24.13215

[7] Sjögren K, Bohlooly Y, Olsson B, Coschigano K, Törnell J, Mohan S, et al. Disproportional skeletal growth and markedly decreased bone mineral content in growth hormone receptor −/− mice. Biochemical and Biophysical Research Communications. 2000;**267**:603-608. DOI: 10.1006/bbrc.1999.1986

[8] Marcovecchio ML, Chiarelly F. Obesity and growth during childhood and puberty. World Review of Nutrition and Dietetics. 2013;**106**:135-141. DOI: 10.1159/000342545

[9] De Leonibus C, Marcovecchio ML, Chiarelli F. Update on statural growth and pubertal development in obese children. Pediatric Reports. 2012;**4**:e35. DOI: 10.4081/pr.2012.e35

[10] Ghione S, Maestro S, Dati E, Silvestri V, Baroncelli GI, Bertelloni S. Growth impairment and growth hormone-IGF-1 axis in infantile anorexia nervosa. Journal of Pediatric Endocrinology & Metabolism. 2015;**28**:999-1001. DOI: 10.1515/jpem-2013-0400

[11] Golden NH, Kreitzer P, Jacobson MS, Chasalow FI, Schebendach J, Freedman SM, et al. Disturbances in growth hormone secretion and action in adolescents with anorexia nervosa. The Journal of Pediatrics. 1994;**125**:655-660

[12] Lazar L, Dan S, Phillip M. Growth without growth hormone: Growth pattern and final height of five patients with idiopathic combined pituitary hormone deficiency. Clinical Endocrinology. 2003;**59**:82-88

[13] Waters MJ, Rowlinson SW, Clarkson RW, Chen CM, Lobie PE, Norstedt G, et al. Signal transduction by the growth hormone receptor. Proceedings of the Society for Experimental Biology and Medicine. 1994;**206**:216-220. DOI: 10.3181/00379727-206-43745

[14] Lobie PE, Mertani H, Morel G, Morales-Bustos O, Norstedt G, Waters MJ. Receptor-mediated nuclear translocation of growth hormone. The Journal of Biological Chemistry. 1994;**269**:21330-21339

[15] Lobie PE, Wood TJ, Chen CM, Waters MJ, Norstedt G. Nuclear translocation and anchorage of the growth hormone receptor. The Journal of Biological Chemistry. 1994;**269**:31735-31746

[16] García-Barros M, Devesa J, Arce VM. Proteolytic processing of human growth hormone (GH) by rat tissues in vitro: Influence of sex and age. Journal of Endocrinological Investigation. 2000;**23**:748-754. DOI: 10.1007/BF03345065

[17] Caicedo D, Díaz O, Devesa P, Devesa J. Growth hormone (GH) and cardiovascular system. International Journal of Molecular Sciences. 2018;**19**. DOI: 10.3390/ijms19010290

[18] Giustina A, Veldhuis JD. Pathophysiology of the neuroregulation of growth hormone secretion in experimental animals and the human. Endocrine Reviews. 1998;**19**:717-797. DOI: 10.1210/edrv.19.6.0353

[19] Pombo M, Castro-Feijóo L. Hormona de crecimiento: dudas razonables después de más de tres décadas de experiencia. Revista Española de Endocrinología Pediátrica. 2010;**1**(Suppl):41-47. DOI: 10.3266/Pulso.ed.RevEspPed2010.vol 1.SupplCongSEEP

[20] Devesa J, Lima L, Lois N, Fraga C, Lechuga MJ, Arce V, et al. Reasons for the variability in growth hormone responses to GHRH challenge: The endogenous hypothalamic-somatotroph rhythm (HSR). Clinical Endocrinology. 1989;**30**:367-377

[21] Devesa J. Clonidine plus GHRH administration for diagnosing growth hormone deficiency in children. Journal of Clinical and Molecular Endocrinology. 2017;**2**:1-6. DOI: 10.21767/2572-5432.10040

[22] Laron Z, Galatzer A. Growth hormone, somatomedin and prolactin—Relationship to brain function. Brain & Development. 1985;**7**:559-567

[23] Lobie PE, Garcia-Aragon J, Lincoln DT, Barnard R, Wilcox JN, Waters MJ. Localization and ontogeny of growth hormone receptor gene expression in the central nervous system. Brain Research. Developmental Brain Research. 1993;**74**:225-233

[24] Nyberg F, Burman P. Growth hormone and its receptors in the central nervous system—Location and functional significance. Hormone Research. 1996;**45**:18-22. DOI: 10.1159/000184753

[25] Root AW. Growth hormone and prolactin in the fetus. Progress in Clinical and Biological Research. 1976;**10**:107-126

[26] Kaplan SL, Grumbach MM, Shepard TH. The ontogenesis of human fetal hormones. I. Growth hormone and insulin. Journal of Clinical Investigation. 1972;**51**:3080-3093

[27] Devesa P, Reimunde P, Gallego R, Devesa J, Arce VM. Growth hormone (GH) treatment may cooperate with locally-produced GH in increasing the proliferative response of hippocampal progenitors to kainate-induced injury. Brain Injury. 2011;**25**:503-510. DOI: 10.3109/02699052.2011.559611

[28] Devesa P, Agasse F, Xapelli S, Almengló C, Devesa J, Malva JO, et al. Growth hormone pathways signaling for cell proliferation and survival in hippocampal neural precursors from postnatal mice. BMC Neuroscience. 2014;**15**:100. DOI: 10.1186/1471-2202-15-100

[29] Lobie PE, Zhu T, Graichen R, Goh EL. Growth hormone, insulin-like growth factor I and the CNS: Localization, function and mechanism of action. Growth Hormone & IGF Research. 2000;**10 Suppl. B**:S1-S6

[30] Pathipati P, Gorba T, Scheepens A, Goffin V, Sun Y, Fraser M. Growth hormone and prolactin regulate human neural stem cell regenerative activity. Neuroscience. 2011;**190**:409-427. DOI: 10.1016/j.neuroscience.2011.05.029

[31] Scheepens A, Williams CE, Breier BH, Guan J, Gluckman PD. A role for the somatotropic axis in neural development, injury and disease. Journal of Pediatric Endocrinology & Metabolism. 2000;**13**(Suppl 6):1483-1491

[32] Heredia M, Fuente A, Criado J, Yajeya J, Devesa J, Riolobos AS. Early growth hormone (GH) treatment promotes relevant motor functional improvement after severe frontal cortex lesion in adult rats. Behavioural Brain Research. 2013;**247**:48-58. DOI: 10.1016/j.bbr.2013.03.012

[33] Alba-Betancourt C, Luna-Acosta JL, Ramírez-Martínez CE, Avila-González D, Granados-Ávalos E, Carranza M, et al. Neuro-protective effects of growth hormone (GH) after hypoxia-ischemia injury in embryonic chicken cerebellum. General and Comparative Endocrinology. 2013;**183**:17-31. DOI: 10.1016/j.ygcen.2012.12.004

[34] Zhang H, Han M, Zhang X, Sun X, Ling F. The effect and mechanisms of growth hormone replacement on cognitive function in rats with traumatic brain injury. PLoS ONE. 2014;**9**:e108518. DOI: 10.1371/journal.pone.0108518

[35] Bhagia V, Gilkison C, Fitts RH, Zgaijardic DJ, High WM Jr, Masel BE, et al. Effect of recombinant growth hormone replacement in a growth hormone deficient subject recovering from mild traumatic brain injury: A case report. Brain Injury. 2010;**24**:560-567. DOI: 10.3109/02699051003601705

[36] High WM Jr, Briones-Galang M, Clark JA, Gilkison C, Mossberg KA, Zgaljardic DJ, et al. Effect of growth hormone replacement therapy on cognition after traumatic brain injury. Journal of Neurotrauma. 2010;**27**:1565-1575. DOI: 10.1089/neu.2009.1253

[37] Maric NP, Doknic M, Pavlovic D, Pekic S, Stojanovic M, Jasovic-Gasic M, et al. Psychiatric and neuropsychological changes in growth hormone-deficient patients after traumatic brain injury in response to growth hormone therapy. Journal of Endocrinological Investigation. 2010;**33**:770-775. DOI: 10.1007/BF03350340

[38] Waters MJ, Blackmore DG. Growth hormone (GH), brain development and neural stem cells. Pediatric Endocrinology Reviews. 2011;**9**:549-553

[39] Reimunde P, Quintana A, Castañón B, Casteleiro N, Vilarnovo Z, Otero A, et al. Effects of growth hormone (GH) replacement and cognitive rehabilitation in patients with

cognitive disorders after traumatic brain injury. Brain Injury. 2011;**25**:65-73. DOI: 10.3109/02699052.2010.536196

[40] Devesa J, Alonso B, Casteleiro N, Couto P, Castañón B, Zas E, et al. Effects of recombinant growth hormone (GH) replacement and psychomotor and cognitive stimulation in the neurodevelopment of GH-deficient (GHD) children with cerebral palsy: A pilot study. Therapeutics and Clinical Risk Management. 2011;**7**:199-206. DOI: 10.2147/TCRM.S21403

[41] Devesa J, Reimunde P, Devesa P, Barbera M, Arce V. Growth hormone (GH) and brain trauma. Hormones and Behavior. 2013;**63**:331-344. DOI: 10.1016/j.yhbeh.2012.02.022

[42] Moreau OK, Cortet-Rudelli C, Yollin E, Merlen E, Daveluy W, Rousseaux M. Growth hormone replacement therapy in patients with traumatic brain injury. Journal of Neurotrauma. 2013;**30**:998-1006. DOI: 10.1089/neu.2012.2705

[43] Arce VM, Devesa P, Devesa J. Role of growth hormone (GH) in the treatment on neural diseases: From neuroprotection to neural repair. Neuroscience Research. 2013;**76**:179-186. DOI: 10.1016/j.neures.2013.03.014

[44] Devesa J, Díaz-Getino G, Rey P, García-Cancela J, Loures I, Nogueiras S, et al. Brain recovery after a plane crash: Treatment with growth hormone (GH) and neurorehabilitation: A case report. International Journal of Molecular Sciences. 2015;**16**:30470-30482. DOI: 10.3390/ijms161226244

[45] Devesa J, Lema H, Zas E, Munín B, Taboada P, Devesa P. Learning and memory recoveries in a young girl treated with growth hormone and neurorehabilitation. Journal of Clinical Medicine. 2016;**5**. DOI: 10.3390/jcm5020014

[46] Bianchi VE, Locatelli V, Rizzi L. Neurotrophic and neuroregenerative effects of GH/IGF1. International Journal of Molecular Sciences. 2017;**18**. DOI: 10.3390/ijms18112441

[47] Dubiel R, Callender L, Dunklin C, Harper C, Bennett M, Kreber L, et al. Phase 2 randomized placebo-controlled clinical trial of recombinant human growth hormone (rhGH) during rehabilitation from traumatic brain injury. Frontiers in Endocrinology (Lausanne). 2018;**9**:520. DOI: 10.3389/fendo.2018.00520

[48] Ong LK, Chow WZ, TeBay C, Kluge M, Pietrogrande G, Zalewska K, et al. Growth hormone improves cognitive function after experimental stroke. Stroke. 2018;**49**:1257-1266. DOI: 10.1161/STROKEAHA.117.020557

[49] Devesa J, Núñez I, Agra C, Bejarano A, Devesa P. Treatment with growth hormone (GH) increased the metabolic activity of the brain in an elder patient not GH-deficient, who suffered mild cognitive alterations and had an ApoE 4/3 genotype. International Journal of Molecular Sciences. 2018;**19**. DOI: 10.3390/ijms19082294

[50] de Bie HMA, Oostrom KJ, Delemarrre-van de Waal HA. Brain development, intelligence and cognitive outcome in children born small for gestational age. Hormone Research in Pædiatrics. 2010;**73**:6-14. DOI: 10.1159/000271911

[51] Noeker M. Neurocognitive development in children experiencing intrauterine growth retardation and born small for gestational age: Pathological, constitutional and therapeutic pathways. Hormone Research. 2005;**64**(Suppl.3):83-88. DOI: 10.1159/000089322

[52] Lister JP, Blatt GJ, DeBassio WA, Kemper TL, Tonkiss J, Galler JR, et al. Effect of protein malnutrition on numbers of neurons in the principal layers of the adult rat hippocampal formation. Hippocampus. 2005;**15**:393-403. DOI: 10.1002/hipo.20065

[53] Mallard C, Loeliger M, Copolov D, Rees S. Reduced number of neurons in the hippocampus and the cerebellum in the postnatal guinea-pig following intrauterine growth-restriction. Neuroscience. 2000;**100**:327-333. DOI: 10.1016/S0306-4522(00)00271-2

[54] Sasaki J, Fukami E, Mimura S, Hayakawa M, Kitoh J, Watanabe K. Abnormal cerebral neuronal migration in a rat model of intrauterine growth retardation induced by synthetic thromboxane A(2). Early Human Development. 2000;**58**:91-99. DOI: 10.1016/S0378-3782(00)00069-4

[55] Mallard EC, Rees S, Stringer M, Cock ML, Harding R. Effects of chronic placental insufficiency on brain development in fetal sheep. Pediatric Research. 1998;**43**:262-270

[56] Dieni S, Rees S. Dendritic morphology is altered in hippocampal neurons following prenatal compromise. Journal of Neurobiology. 2003;**55**:41-52. DOI: 10.1002/neu.10194

[57] Hayakawa M, Mimura S, Sasaki J, Watanabe K. Neuropathological changes in the cerebrum of IUGR rat induced by synthetic thromboxane A2. Early Human Development. 1999;**55**:125-136. DOI: 10.1016/S0378-3782(99)00023-7

[58] Tashima L, Nakata M, Anno K, Sugino N, Kato H. Prenatal influence of ischemia-hypoxia-induced intrauterine growth retardation on brain development and behavioral activity in rats. Biology of the Neonate. 2000;**80**:81-87. DOI: 10.1159/000047125

[59] Nitsos I, Rees S. The effects of intrauterine growth retardation on the development of the neuroglia in fetal guinea pigs. An immunohistochemical and an ultrastructural study. International Journal of Developmental Neuroscience. 1990;**8**:233-244. DOI: 10.1016/0736-5748(90)90029-2

[60] Sizonenko SV, Borradori-Tolsa C, Bauthay DM, Lodygensky G, Lazeyras F, Huppi P. Impact of intrauterine growth restriction and glucocorticoids on brain development: Insights using advanced magnetic resonance imaging. Molecular and Cellular Endocrinology. 2006;**254-255**:163-171. DOI: 10.1016/j.mce.2006.04.035

[61] Dubois J, Benders M, Borradori-Tolsa C, Cachia A, Lazeyras F, Ha-Vinh LR, et al. Primary cortical folding in the human newborn: an early marker of later functional development. Brain. 2008;**13**:2028-2041. DOI: 10.1093/brain/awn137

[62] Tolsa CB, Zimine S, Warfield SK, Freschi M, Sancho RA, Lazeyras F, et al. Early alteration of structural and functional brain development in premature infants born with

intrauterine growth restriction. Pediatric Research. 2004;**56**:132-138. DOI: 10.1203/01.PDR.0000128983.54614.7E

[63] Toft PB, Leth H, Ring PB, Peitersen B, Lou HC, Henriksen O. Volumetric analysis of the normal infant brain and in intrauterine growth retardation. Early Human Development. 1995;**43**:15-29. DOI: 10.1016/0378-3782(95)01657-O

[64] Arwert LI, Veltman DJ, Deijen JB, van Dam PS, Delemarre-van deWaal HA, Drent ML. Growth hormone deficiency and memory functioning in adults visualized by functional magnetic resonance imaging. Neuroendocrinology. 2005;**82**:32-40. DOI: 10.1159/000090123

[65] Chaplin JE, Kriström B, Jonsson B, Hägglöf B, Tuvemo T, Aronson AS, et al. Improvements in behaviour and self-esteem following growth hormone treatment in short prepubertal children. Hormone Research in Paediatrics. 2011;**75**:291-303. DOI: 10.1159/000322937

[66] Geisler A, Lass N, Reinsch N, Uysal Y, Singer V, Ravens-Sieberer U, et al. Quality of life in children and adolescents with growth hormone deficiency: Association with growth hormone treatment. Hormone Research in Pædiatrics. 2012;**78**:94-99. DOI: 10.1159/000341151

[67] Deijen JB, de Boer H, Blok GJ, van der Veen EA. Cognitive impairments and mood disturbances in growth hormone deficient men. Psychoneuroendocrinology. 1996;**21**:313-322. DOI: 10.1016/0306-4530(95)00050-X

[68] McGauley G, Cuneo R, Salomon F, Sönksen PH. Growth hormone deficiency and quality of life. Hormone Research. 1996;**45**:34-37. DOI: 10.1159/000184756

[69] Falleti MG, Maruff P, Burman P, Harris A. The effects of growth hormone (GH) deficiency and GH replacement on cognitive performance in adults: A meta-analysis of the current literature. Psychoneuroendocrinology. 2006;**31**:681-691. DOI: 10.1016/j.psyneuen.2006.01.005

[70] Nyberg F, Hallberg M. Growth hormone and cognitive function. Nature Reviews. Endocrinology. 2013;**9**:357-365. DOI: 10.1038/nrendo.2013.78

[71] Rosén T, Wirén L, Wilhelmsen L, Wiklund I, Bengtsson BA. Decreased psychological well-being in adult patients with growth hormone deficiency. Clinical Endocrinology. 1994;**40**:111-116. DOI: 10.1111/j.1365-2265.1994.tb02452.x

[72] Li E, Kim DH, Cai M, Lee S. Hippocampus-dependent spatial learning and memory are impaired in growth hormone-deficient spontaneous dwarf rats. Endocrine Journal. 2011;**58**:257-267. DOI: 10.1507/endocrj.K11E-006

[73] Bevan P. Insulin signaling. Journal of Cell Science. 2001;**114**:1429-1430. ISSN: 0021-9533

[74] Le Grevés M, Zhou Q, Berg M, Le Grevés P, Fhölenhag K, Meyerson B, et al. Growth hormone replacement in hypophysectomized rats affects spatial performance and

hippocampal levels of NMDA receptor subunit and PSD-95 gene transcript levels. Experimental Brain Research. 2006;**173**:267-273. DOI: 10.1007/s00221-006-0438-2

[75] Park SW, Shin S, Kim CH, Ko AR, Kwak MJ, Nam MH, et al. Differential effects of insufflated, subcutaneous, and intravenous growth hormone on bone growth, cognitive function, and NMDA receptor subunit expression. Endocrinology. 2010;**151**:4418-4427. DOI: 10.1210/en.2010-0152

[76] Le Grevès M, Steensland P, Le Grevès P, Nyberg F. Growth hormone induces age-dependent alteration in the expression of hippocampal growth hormone receptor and N-methyl-D-aspartate receptor subunits gene transcripts in male rats. Proceedings of the National Academy of Sciences of the United States of America. 2002;**99**:7119-7123. DOI: 10.1073/pnas.092135399

[77] Mahmoud GS, Grover LM. Growth hormone enhances excitatory synaptic transmission in area CA1 of rat hippocampus. Journal of Neurophysiology. 2006;**95**:2962-2974. DOI: 10.1152/jn.00947.2005

[78] Devesa J, Casteleiro N, Rodicio C, López N, Reimunde P. Growth hormone deficiency and cerebral palsy. Therapeutics and Clinical Risk Management. 2010;**6**:413-418. DOI: 10.2147/tcrm.s12312

[79] Reimunde P, Rodicio C, López N, Alonso A, Devesa P, Devesa J. Effects of growth hormone replacement and physical rehabilitation in recovery of gross motor function in children with cerebral palsy. Therapeutics and Clinical Risk Management. 2010;**6**:585-592. DOI: 10.2147/TCRM.S14919

[80] Song J, Park K, Lee H, Kim M. The effect of recombinant human growth hormone therapy in patients with completed stroke: A pilot trial. Annals of Rehabilitation Medicine. 2012;**36**:447-457. DOI: 10.5535/arm.2012.36.4.447

[81] Quintana A, Agra C, Outeiral L, Devesa A, Llorente D, Devesa J. Cognitive evolution of a patient who suffered a subarachnoid haemorrhage eight years ago, after being treated with growth hormone, melatonin and neurorehabilitation. Report. 2018;**1**:2-16. DOI: 10.3390/reports1010002

[82] Devesa J, López Segade N, Isorna J, Devesa P, Castellanos S, Puell CI. Is the use of growth hormone and melatonin justified in spinal cord injuries? MOJ Anatomy & Physiology. 2017;**4**:258-262. DOI: 10.15406/mojap.2017.04.00128

[83] Shetty KR, Sutton CH, Mattson DE, Rudman D. Hyposomatomedinemia in quadriplegic men. The American Journal of the Medical Sciences. 1993;**305**:95-100. DOI: 10.1097/00000441-199302000-00006

[84] Bauman WA, Spungen AM, Flanagan S, Zhong YG, Alexander LR, Tsitouras PD. Blunted growth hormone response to intravenous arginine in subjects with a spinal cord injury. Hormone and Metabolic Research. 1994;**26**:152-156. DOI: 10.1055/s-2007-1000798

[85] Cuatrecasas G, Kumru H, Coves MJ, Vidal J. GH deficiency in patients with spinal cord injury: Efficacy/safety of GH replacement, a pilot study. Endocrine Connections. 2018;**7**:1031-1039. DOI: 10.1530/EC-18-0296

[86] Devesa J, Alonso A, López N, García J, Puell CI, Pablos T, et al. Growth hormone (GH) and rehabilitation promoted distal innervation in a child affected by caudal regression syndrome. International Journal of Molecular Sciences. 2017;**18**. DOI: 10.3390/ijms18010230

[87] Attias J, Zarchi O, Nageris BI, Laron Z. Cochlear hearing loss in patients with Laron syndrome. European Archives of Oto-Rhino-Laryngology. 2012;**269**:461-466. DOI: 10.1007/s00405-011-1668-x

[88] Muus J, Weir F, Kreicher K. Hearing loss in children with growth hormone deficiency. International Journal of Pediatric Otorhinolaryngology. 2017;**100**:107-113. DOI: 10.1016/j.ijporl.2017.06.037

[89] Guerra J, Devesa A, Llorente D, Mouro R, Alonso A, García-Cancela J, et al. Early treatment with growth hormone (GH) and rehabilitation recovers hearing in a child with cerebral palsy. Report. 2019;**2**:4-12. DOI: 10.3390/reports2010004

[90] Devesa J, Devesa P, Reimunde P, Arce V. Growth hormone and kynesitherapy for brain injury recovery. In: Agrawal A, editor. Brain Injury—Pathogenesis, Monitoring, Recovery and Management. London, United Kingdom: IntechOpen; 2012. pp. 417-454. DOI: 10.5772/26998.ch21

[91] Devesa J, Reimunde P, Devesa A, Souto S, López-Amado M, Devesa P, et al. Recovery from neurological sequelae secondary to oncological brain surgery in an adult growth hormone-deficient after growth hormone treatment. Journal of Rehabilitation Medicine. 2009;**41**:775-777. DOI: 10.2340/16501977-0416

[92] Devesa P, Gelabert M, González-Mosquera T, Gallego R, Relova JL, Devesa J, et al. Growth hormone treatment enhances the functional recovery of sciatic nerves after transection and repair. Muscle & Nerve. 2012;**45**:385-392. DOI: 10.1002/mus.22303

[93] Saccà L, Cittadini A, Fazio S. Growth hormone and the heart. Endocrine Reviews. 1994;**5**:555-573. DOI: 10.1210/edrv-15-5-555

[94] Li Q, Li B, Wang X, Leri A, Jana KP, Liu Y, et al. Overexpression of insulin-like growth factor-I in mice protects from myocyte death after infarction, attenuating ventricular dilation, wall stress, and cardiac hypertrophy. The Journal of Clinical Investigation. 1997;**100**:1991-1999. DOI: 10.1172/JCI119730

[95] Timsit J, Riou B, Bertherat J, Wisnewsky C, Kato NS, Weisberg AS, et al. Effects of chronic growth hormone hypersecretion on intrinsic contractility, energetics, isomyosin pattern, and myosin adenosine triphosphatase activity of rat left ventricle. The Journal of Clinical Investigation. 1990;**86**:507-515. DOI: 10.1172/JCI114737

[96] Cittadini A, Ishiguro Y, Strömer H, Spindler M, Moses AC, Clark R, et al. Insulin-like growth factor-1 but not growth hormone augments mammalian myocardial contractility by sensitizing the myofilament to Ca2+ through a wortmannin-sensitive pathway: studies in rat and ferret isolated muscles. Circulation Research. 1998;**83**:50-59. DOI: 10.1161/01.res.83.1.50

[97] Buerke M, Murohara T, Skurk C, Nuss C, Tomaselli K, Lefer AM. Cardioprotective effect of insulin-like growth factor I in myocardial ischemia followed by reperfusion. Proceedings of the National Academy of Sciences of the United States of America. 1995;**92**:8031-8035. DOI: 10.1073/pnas.92.17.8031

[98] Ren J. Short-term administration of insulin-like growth factor (IGF-1) does not induce myocardial IGF-1 resistance. Growth Hormone & IGF Research. 2002;**12**:162-168. DOI: 10.1016/S1096-6374(02)00020-5

[99] Brüel A, Oxlund H. Biosynthetic growth hormone increase the collagen deposition rate in rat aorta and heart. European Journal of Endocrinology. 1995;**132**:195-199. DOI: 10.1530/eje.0.1320195

[100] Longobardi S, Cuocolo A, Merola B, Di Rella F, Colao A, Nicolai E, et al. Left ventricular function in young adults with childhood and adulthood onset growth hormone deficiency. Clinical Endocrinology. 1998;**48**:137-143. DOI: 10.1046/j.1365-2265.1998.00281.x

[101] Thuesen L, Jorgensen JO, Müller JR, Kristensen BO, Skakkebaek NE, Vahl N, et al. Short and long-term cardiovascular effects of growth hormone deficient adults. Clinical Endocrinology. 1994;**41**:615-650. DOI: 10.1111/j.1365-2265.1994.tb01827.x

[102] Valcavi R, Gaddi O, Zini M, Iavicoli M, Mellino U, Portioli I. Cardiac performance and mass in adult with hypopituitarism: Effects of one year of growth treatment. The Journal of Clinical Endocrinology and Metabolism. 1995;**80**:659-666. DOI: 10.1210/jcem.80.2.7852533

[103] Johannsson G, Bengtsson BA, Andersson B, Isgaard J, Caidahl K. Long-term cardiovascular effects of growth hormone treatment in GH-deficient adults: Preliminary data in a small group of patients. Clinical Endocrinology. 1996;**45**:305-314. DOI: 10.1046/j.1365-2265.1996.00820.x

[104] Cuneo RC, Salomon F, Wiles CM, Hesp R, Sönksen PH. Growth hormone treatment in growth hormone deficient adults. I. Effects on muscle mass and strength. Journal of Applied Physiology. 1991;**70**:688-694. DOI: 10.1152/jappl.1991.70.2.688

[105] Cuneo RC, Salomon F, Wiles CM, Hesp R, Sönksen PH. Growth hormone treatment in growth hormone-deficient adults. II. Effects on exercise performance. Journal of Applied Physiology. 1991;**70**:695-700. DOI: 10.1152/jappl.1991.70.2.695

[106] Colao A, Cuocolo A, Di Somma C, Cerbone G, Della Morte AM, Nicolai E, et al. Impaired cardiac performance in elderly patients with growth hormone deficiency. The Journal of Clinical Endocrinology and Metabolism. 1999;**85**:3950-3955. DOI: 10.1210/jcem.84.11.6112

[107] Colao A, Di Somma C, Cuocolo A, Filipella M, Rota F, Acampa W, et al. The severity of GH deficiency (GHD) correlates with the severity of cardiac impairment in 100 adult patients with hypopituitarism: An observational, case-control study. The Journal of Clinical Endocrinology and Metabolism. 2004;**89**:5998-6004. DOI: 10.1210/jc.2004-1042

[108] Maison P, Chanson P. Cardiac effects of growth hormone in adults with growth hormone deficiency. Circulation. 2003;**108**:2648-2652. DOI: 10.1161/01.CIR.0000100720.01867.1D

[109] Isgaard J, Arcopinto M, Karason K, Cittadini A. GH and the cardiovascular system: An update on a topic at heart. Endocrine. 2015;**48**:25-35. DOI: 10.1007/s12020-014-0327-6

[110] Thomas JD, Dattani A, Zemrak F, Burchell T, Akker SA, Gurnell M, et al. Characterisation of myocardial structure and function in adult-onset growth hormone deficiency using cardiac magnetic resonance. Endocrine. 2016;**54**:778-787. DOI: 10.1007/s12020-016-1067-6

[111] Capalbo D, Barbieri F, Improda N, Giallauria F, Di Pietro E, Rapacciuolo A, et al. Growth hormone improves cardiopulmonary capacity and body composition in children with growth hormone deficiency. The Journal of Clinical Endocrinology and Metabolism. 2017;**102**:4080-4088. DOI: 10.1210/jc.2017-00871

[112] Cittadini A, D'Assante R. Growth hormone in heart failure revisited: An old story retold. Monaldi Archives for Chest Disease. 2018;**88**:989. DOI: 10.4081/monaldi.2018.989

[113] Salzano A, Marra AM, D'Assante R, Arcopinto M, Suzuki T, Bossone E, et al. Growth hormone therapy in heart failure. Heart Failure Clinics. 2018;**14**:501-515. DOI: 10.1016/j.hfc.2018.05.002

[114] Arcopinto M, Salzano A, Giallauria F, Bossone E, Isgaard J, Marra AM, et al. Growth hormone deficiency is associated with worse cardiac function, physical performance, and outcome in chronic heart failure: Insights from the T.O.S.CA. GHD study. PLoS ONE. 2017;**12**:e0170058. DOI: 10.1371/journal.pone.0170058

[115] Gómez-Guzmán E, Cañete MD, Valle-Martos R, Cañete R, Valle M, Jiménez-Reina L, et al. Short-term evaluation of left ventricular mass and function in children with growth hormone deficiency after replacement treatment. Frontiers in Pediatrics. 2018;**6**:174. DOI: 10.3389/fped.2018.00174

[116] Marra AM, Bobbio E, D'Assante R, Salzano A, Arcopinto M, Bossone E, et al. Growth hormone as biomarker in heart failure. Heart Failure Clinics. 2018;**14**:65-74. DOI: 10.1016/j.hfc.2017.08.008

[117] Piccioli L, Arcopinto M, Salzano A, D'Assante R, Schiavo A, Stagnaro FM, et al. The impairment of the growth hormone/insulin-like growth factor 1 (IGF-1) axis in heart failure: A possible target for future therapy. Monaldi Archives for Chest Disease. 2018;**88**:975. DOI: 10.4081/monaldi.2018.975

[118] Ziagaki A, Blaschke D, Haverkamp W, Plöckinger U. Long-term growth hormone (GH)-replacement of adult GH-deficiency (GHD) benefits the heart. European Journal of Endocrinology. 2019. DOI: 10.1530/EJE-19-0132

[119] Wang T, Liu J, McDonald C, Lupino K, Zhai X, Wilkins BJ, et al. GDF15 is a heart-derived hormone that regulates body growth. EMBO Molecular Medicine. 2017;**9**:1150-1164. DOI: 10.15252/emmm.201707604

[120] Walsh MF, Barazi M, Pete G, Muniyappa R, Dunbar JC, Sowers JR. Insulin-like growth factor I diminishes *in vivo* and *in vitro* vascular contractility: role of vascular nitric oxide. Endocrinology. 1996;**137**:1798-1803. DOI: 10.1210/endo.137.5.8612517

[121] Tsukahara H, Gordienko DV, Tonshoff B, Gelato MC, Goligorsky MS. Direct demonstration of insulin-like growth factor-I-induced nitric oxide production by endothelial cells. Kidney International. 1994;**45**:598-604. DOI: 10.1038/ki.1994.78

[122] Muniyappa R, Walsh MF, Rangi JS, et al. Insulin like growth factor 1 increases vascular smooth muscle nitric oxide production. Life Sciences. 1997;**61**:925-931. DOI: 10.1016/s0024-3205(97)00594-8

[123] Haylor J, Singh I, Nahas AM. Nitric oxide synthesis inhibitor prevents vasodilation by insulin-like growth factor I. Kidney International. 1991;**39**:333-335. DOI: 10.1038/ki.1991.42

[124] Napoli R, Guardasole V, Matarazzo M, Palmieri EA, Oliviero U, Fazio S, et al. Growth hormone corrects vascular dysfunction in patients with chronic heart failure. Journal of the American College of Cardiology. 2002;**39**:90-95. DOI: 10.1016/S0735-1097(01)01707-7

[125] Capaldo B, Guardasole V, Pardo F, Matarazzo M, Di Rella F, Numis F, et al. Abnormal vascular reactivity in growth hormone deficiency. Circulation. 2001;**103**:520-524. DOI: 10.1161/01.cir.103.4.520

[126] Tivesten A, Barlind A, Caidahl K, Klintland N, Cittadini A, Ohlsson C, et al. Growth hormone-induced blood pressure decrease is associated with increased mRNA levels of the vascular smooth muscle KATP channel. The Journal of Endocrinology. 2004;**183**:195-202. DOI: 10.1677/joe.1.05726

[127] Suzuki K, Yanagi K, Shimizu M, Wakamatsu S, Niitani T, Hosonuma S, et al. Effect of growth hormone replacement therapy on plasma diacron-reactive oxygen metabolites and endothelial function in Japanese patients: The GREAT clinical study. Endocrine Journal. 2018;**65**:101-111. DOI: 10.1507/endocrj.EJ17-0330

[128] Sverrisdóttir Y, Elam M, Bengtsson B-Å, Johannsson G. Intense sympathetic nerve activity in adults with hypopituitarism and untreated growth hormone deficiency. The Journal of Clinical Endocrinology and Metabolism. 1998;**83**:1881-1885. DOI: 10.1210/jcem.83.6.4895

[129] Sverrisdóttir Y, Elam M, Caidahl K, Söderling AS, Herlitz H, Johannsson G. The effect of growth hormone (GH) replacement therapy on sympathetic nerve hyperactivity in hypopituitary adults: A double-blind, placebo-controlled, cross-over, short-term trial followed by long-term open GH replacement in hypopituitary adults. Journal of Hypertension. 2003;**10**:1905-1914. DOI: 10.1097/01.jhj.000084757.37215.55

[130] Oomen PH, Beentjes JA, Bosma E, Smit AJ, Reitsma WD, Dullaart RP. Reduced capillary permeability and capillary density in the skin of GH-deficient adults: Improvement after 12 months GH replacement. Clinical Endocrinology (Oxf). 2002;**56**:519-524. DOI: 10.1046/j.1365-2265.2002.01517.x

[131] Hellstrom A, Svensson E, Carlsson B, Niklasson A, Albertsson-Wikland K. Reduced retinal vascularization in children with growth hormone deficiency. The Journal of Clinical Endocrinology and Metabolism. 1999;**84**:795-798. DOI: 10.1210/jcem.84.2.5484

[132] Hellstrom A, Carlsson B, Niklasson A, Segnestam K, Boguszewski M, de Lacerda L, et al. IGF-I is critical for normal vascularization of the human retina. The Journal of Clinical Endocrinology and Metabolism. 2002;**87**:3413-3416. DOI: 10.1210/jcem.87.7.8629

[133] Castellano G, Affuso F, Di Conza P, Fazio S. The GH/IGF-I axis and heart failure. Current Cardiology Reviews. 2009;**5**:203-215. DOI: 10.2174/157340309788970306

[134] Clapp C, Thebault S, Jeziorski MC, Martínez de la Escalera G. Peptide hormone regulation of angiogenesis. Physiological Reviews. 2009;**89**:1177-1215. DOI: 10.1152/physrev.00024.2009

[135] Bartlett JM, Charlton HM, Robinson IC, Nieschlag E. Pubertal development and testicular function in the male growth hormone-deficient rat. The Journal of Endocrinology. 1990;**126**:193-201. DOI: 10.1677/joe.0.1260193

[136] Hull KL, Harvey S. Growth hormone: Roles in male reproduction. Endocrine. 2000;**13**:243-250. DOI: 10.1385/ENDO:13:3:243

[137] Martínez-Moreno CG, López-Marín LM, Carranza M, Giterman D, Harvey S, Arámburo C, et al. Growth hormone (GH) and GH-releasing hormone (GHRH): Co-localization and action in the chicken testis. General and Comparative Endocrinology. 2014;**199**:38-45. DOI: 10.1016/j.ygcen.2014.01.013

[138] Berensztein EB, Baquedano MS, Pepe CM, Constanzo M, Saraco NI, Ponzio R, et al. Role of IGFs and insulin in the human testis during postnatal activation: Differentiation of steroidogenic cells. Pediatric Research. 2008;**63**:662-666. DOI: 10.1203/PDR.0b013e3186c8ffc

[139] Gallego R, Pintos E, García-Caballero T, Raghay K, Boulanger L, Beiras A, et al. Cellular distribution of growth hormone releasing hormone receptor in human reproductive system and breast and prostate cancers. Histology and Histopathology. 2005;**20**:697-706. DOI: 10.14670/HH-20.697

[140] Tena-Sempere M. Exploring the role of ghrelin as novel regulator of gonadal function. Growth Hormone & IGF Research. 2005;**15**:83-88. DOI: 19.1016/j.ghir.2005.02.001

[141] Riaz H, Liang A, Khan MK, Dong P, Han L, Shahzad M, et al. Somatostatin and its receptors: Functional regulation in the development of mice Sertoli cells. The Journal of Steroid Biochemistry and Molecular Biology. 2013;**138**:257-266. DOI: 10.1016/j.jsbmb.2013.06.007

[142] Nguyen AP, Chandorkar A, Gupta C. The role of growth hormone in fetal mouse reproductive tract differentiation. Endocrinology. 1996;**137**:3659-3666. DOI: 10.1210/endo.137.9.8756530

[143] Laron Z, Klinger B. Effect of insulin-like growth factor-I treatment on serum androgens and testicular and penile size in males with Laron syndrome (primary growth

hormone resistance). European Journal of Endocrinology. 1998;**138**:176-180. DOI: 10.1530/eje.0.1380176

[144] Carani C, Granata ARM, De Rosa M, Garau C, Zarrili S, Paesano L, et al. The effect of chronic treatment with GH on gonadal function in men with isolated GH deficiency. European Journal of Endocrinology. 1999;**140**:224-230. DOI: 10.1530/eje.0.1400224

[145] Balducci R, Toscano V, Mangiantini A, Bianchi P, Guglielmi R, Boscherini B. The effect of growth hormone administration on testicular response during gonadotropin therapy in subjects with combined gonadotropin and growth hormone deficiencies. Acta Endocrinology (Copenh). 1993;**128**:19-23. DOI: 10.1530/acta.0.1280019

[146] Tatò L, Zamboni G, Antoniazzi F, Piubello G. Gonadal function and response to growth hormone (GH) in boys with isolated GH deficiency and to GH and gonadotropins in boys with multiple pituitary hormone deficiencies. Fertility and Sterility. 1996;**65**:830-834. DOI: 10.1016/s0015-0282(16)58222-3

[147] Oscarsson J, Lindstedt G, Lundberg PA, Edén S. Continuous subcutaneous infusion of low dose growth hormone decreases serum sex-hormone binding globulin and testosterone concentrations in moderately obese middle-aged men. Clinical Endocrinology (Oxf). 1996;**44**:23-29. DOI: 10.1046/j.1365-2265.1996.635457.x

[148] Giavoli C, Ferrante E, Ermetici F, Bergamaschi S, Ronchi CL, Lania AG, et al. Effect of recombinant hGH (rhGH) replacement on gonadal function in male patients with organic adult-onset GH deficiency. Clinical Endocrinology. 2006;**65**:717-721. DOI: 10.1111/j.1365-2265.2006.02655.x

[149] Andreassen M, Frystyk J, Faber J, Kristensen LØ, Juul A. Growth hormone (GH) activity is associated with increased serum oestradiol and reduced Anti-Müllerian Hormone in healthy male volunteers treated with GH and a GH antagonist. Andrology. 2013;**1**:595-601. DOI: 10.1111/j.2047-2927.2013.00096.x

[150] Boonstra VH, Weber RF, de Jong FH, Hokken-Koelega AC. Hormone Research. 2008;**70**:357-363. DOI: 10.1159/000161866

[151] Silveira MA, Zampieri TT, Furigo IC, Abdulkader F, Donato J Jr, Frazan R. Acute effects of somatomammotropin hormones on neuronal components of the hypothalamic-pituitary-gonadal axis. Brain Research. 1714;**2019**:210-217. DOI: 10.1016/j.brainres.2019.03.003

[152] Untergasser G, Hermann M, Rumpold H, Berger P. Complex alternative splicing of the GH-V gene in the human testis. European Journal of Endocrinology. 1998;**1394**:424-427. DOI: 10.1530/eje.0.1390424

[153] Luna M, Martínez-Moreno CG, Ahumada-Solórzano MS, Harvey S, Carranza M, Arámburo C. Extrapituitary growth hormone in the chicken reproductive system. General and Comparative Endocrinology. 2014;**203**:60-68. DOI: 10.1016/j.ygcen.2014.02.021

[154] Ménézo YJ, Nicollet B, Rollet J, Hazout A. Pregnancy and delivery after in vitro maturation of naked ICSI-GV oocytes with GH and transfer of a frozen thawed blastocyst: Case report. Journal of Assisted Reproduction and Genetics. 2006;**23**:47-49. DOI: 10.1007/s10815-005-9014-0

[155] Shirazi A, Shams-Esfandabadi N, Ahmadi E, Heidari B. Effects of growth hormone on nuclear maturation of ovine oocytes and subsequent embryo development. Reproduction in Domestic Animals. 2010;**45**:530-536. DOI: 10.1111/j.1439-0531.2008.01290.x

[156] Lobie PE, Breipohl W, Aragón JG, Waters MJ. Cellular localization of the growth hormone receptor/binding protein in the male and female reproductive systems. Endocrinology. 1990;**126**:2214-2221. DOI: 10.1210/endo-126-4-2214

[157] Abir R, Garor R, Felz C, Nitke S, Krissi H, Fisch B. Growth hormone and its receptor in human ovaries from fetuses and adults. Fertility and Sterility. 2008;**90**:1333-1339. DOI: 10.1016/j.fertnstert.2007.08.011

[158] De Prada JK, VandeVoort CA. Growth hormone and in vitro maturation of rhesus macaque oocytes and subsequent embryo development. Journal of Assisted Reproduction and Genetics. 2008;**25**:145-158. DOI: 10.1007/s10815-008-9208-3

[159] Izadyar F, Hage WJ, Colenbrander B, Bevers MM. The promotory effect of growth hormone on the developmental competence of in vitro matured bovine oocytes is due to improved cytoplasmic maturation. Molecular Reproduction and Development. 1998;**49**:444-453. DOI: 10.1002/(SICI)1098-2795(199804)49:4<444::AID-MRD12>3.0.CO:2-U

[160] Hull KL, Harvey S. Growth hormone: Roles in female reproduction. The Journal of Endocrinology. 2001;**168**:1-23. DOI: 10.1155/2014/234014

[161] Wilson ME. The impact of the GH-IGF-I axis on gonadotropin secretion: Inferences from animal models. Journal of Pediatric Endocrinology & Metabolism. 2001;**14**:115-140. DOI: 10.1515/JPEM.2001.14.2.115

[162] Chandrashekar V, Zaczek D, Bartke A. The consequences of altered somatotropic system on reproduction. Biology of Reproduction. 2004;**71**:17-27. DOI: 10.1095/biolreprod.103.027060

[163] Spiliotis BE. Growth hormone insufficiency and its impact on ovarian function. Annals of the New York Academy of Sciences. 2003;**997**:77-84. DOI: 10.1196/annals.1290.009

[164] Giampietro A, Milardi D, Bianchi A, Fusco A, Cimino V, Valle D, et al. The effect of treatment with growth hormone on fertility outcome in eugonadal women with growth hormone deficiency: Report of four cases and review of the literature. Fertility and Sterility. 2009;**91**:390.e7-11. DOI: 10.1016/j.fertnstert.2008.09.065

[165] Sharara FI, Giudice LC. Role of growth hormone in ovarian physiology and onset of puberty. Journal of the Society for Gynecologic Investigation. 1997;**4**:2-7. DOI: 10.1016/S1071-5576(96)00059-7

[166] Lee M. Growth hormone deficiency as the only identifiable cause for primary amenorrhea. Journal of Pediatric and Adolescent Gynecology. 2000;**13**:93. DOI: 10.1016/S1083-3188(00)00025-5

[167] Devesa J, Caicedo D. The role of growth hormone on ovarian functioning and ovarian angiogenesis. Frontiers in Endocrinology. 2019;**10**:450. DOI: 10.3389/fendo.2019.00450

[168] Cui N, Li AM, Luo ZY, Zhao ZM, Xu YM, Zhang J, et al. Effects of growth hormone on pregnancy rates of patients with thin endometrium. Journal of Endocrinological Investigation. 2019;**42**:27-35. DOI: 10.1007/s40618-018-0877-1

[169] Markham KE, Kaye PL. Growth hormone, insulin-like growth factor I and cell proliferation in the mouse blastocyst. Reproduction. 2003;**125**:327-336. DOI: 10.1007/s40618-018-0877-1

[170] Vila G, Luger A. Growth hormone deficiency and pregnancy: Any role for substitution? Minerva Endocrinologica. 2018;**43**:451-457. DOI: 10.23736/S0391-1977.18.02834-1

Chapter 3

Growth Hormone Deficiency: Is It Just a Problem of Growth Impairment? Part II

Jesús Devesa

Additional information is available at the end of the chapter

http://dx.doi.org/10.5772/intechopen.89159

Abstract

As stated in the first part of this review, growth hormone (GH) acts on all organs and tissues, and untreated GH-deficient (GHD) patients suffer from several affectations occurring as a consequence of the lack of this key hormone. In the second part of this review, we will analyze the effects of GH on the liver, the kidney, the adrenal glands, the skeletal muscles, the bones, the hematopoietic system, the gastrointestinal system, and the adverse effects that may occur in these organs and systems in the GH deficiency not treated in children and adults. Apart from these, we conclude that GH is a co-hormone that seems to be necessary for the physiological actions of other important hormones in humans.

Keywords: GH deficiency, IGF-I, GH and liver, GH and kidney, GH and adipose tissue, GH and the hematopoietic system, GH and skeletal muscles

1. Introduction

GH, many times directly, and in other cases by cooperating with other hormones, or acting through its own mediators, plays a role in the regeneration of the liver, in the development and normal functioning of the kidney, in the amount of fat mass, in the development and maintenance of skeletal muscles, in the skeletal development and mineral acquisition in bones, and in systems as complex as the hematopoietic system and the immune system; in addition, the hormone is able to act at the gastrointestinal level and also on the adrenal glands. In this second part of this review, we will analyze the physiological effects of the hormone on these organs and systems, as well as the consequences of its loss when it is untreated with replacement therapy.

IntechOpen

© 2019 The Author(s). Licensee IntechOpen. This chapter is distributed under the terms of the Creative Commons Attribution License (http://creativecommons.org/licenses/by/3.0), which permits unrestricted use, distribution, and reproduction in any medium, provided the original work is properly cited. (cc) BY

1.1. GHD and liver

The liver is an important organ, where the actions of GH take place. For instance, the loss of critical GH signaling pathways in mice with liver-specific knockouts leads these animals to share a common phenotype of hepatic steatosis [1–3], indicating that GH plays an important physiological role in hepatic triglyceride metabolism. Steatosis leads to hepatic degeneration, which may be corrected by GH administration. A high prevalence of liver dysfunction has been reported in adult GHD patients [4], while GH-replacement therapy significantly reduced serum liver enzyme concentrations in these patients and improved the histological changes in their fatty liver [4–7]. Clinical reports in children have shown the same association between untreated GHD and liver steatosis [8–12], which is recovered after GH-replacement therapy. These effects of GH on liver repair are curious because the liver produces its own factor of regeneration: hepatocyte growth factor (HGF), first identified in the sera of 70% hepatectomized rats, as a mitogen of adult rat hepatocytes [13, 14]. Animal studies, using either anti-HGF antibody or *c-Met* gene destruction techniques, revealed that both the endocrine and paracrine effects of HGF are involved in liver growth after 70% hepatectomy and for recovery from hepatitis, respectively [15–18]. In spite of its liver production and its strong liver regenerative properties, it was found that in hypophysectomized rats, the responses of hepatic HGF gene expression and DNA synthesis to partial hepatectomy were accelerated by treatment with GH [19]. Whether GH stimulates the transcription of HGF or facilitates, it is not known, but our group found that GH is expressed in the liver of hypophysectomized rats subjected to partial hepatectomy and that this GH promotes the hepatic regeneration, directly or via HGF induction [20]. In this study, the analysis of the products obtained with the enzyme of restriction RsaI demonstrated that the hepatic GH gives origin to two bands in the expected molecular weight position (238 and 90 bp), identical to the bands obtained from pituitary rat GH [20]; see Figure 7 for this reference. From these data, it is clear that there is a hepatic expression of GH that contributes to, or determines, the high degree of regenerating ability of the liver, apart from playing important metabolic functions in this organ. As suggested above in the case of testis in GHD patients, it would be interesting to investigate whether the hepatic expression of GH exists or not in untreated GHD humans. In any case, GH-replacement therapy plays an important reparative function in non-alcoholic liver steatosis, and perhaps in other liver diseases (**Figure 1**).

1.2. GHD and kidney

GH exerts important effects on the kidney, affecting renal function and kidney growth. GHR mRNA expression has been found in rat kidney during fetal development and adulthood [21]. This GHR expression was found in all nephron segments, with the strongest signals in the distal convoluted tubule and the collecting duct and a very weak signal in the glomeruli [22]. GHR expression has also been found in human fetal kidneys as early as 8.5–9 weeks of gestation [23]. GHR expression was stronger in the outer medulla than in the cortex and remained similar at midgestation and after birth. The fact that weak staining was also found in immature glomeruli in early gestation but disappeared at later developmental stages [23] suggests that GH is involved in glomerular morphogenesis. The kidney expression of GHR

http://dx.doi.org/10.5772/intechopen.89159

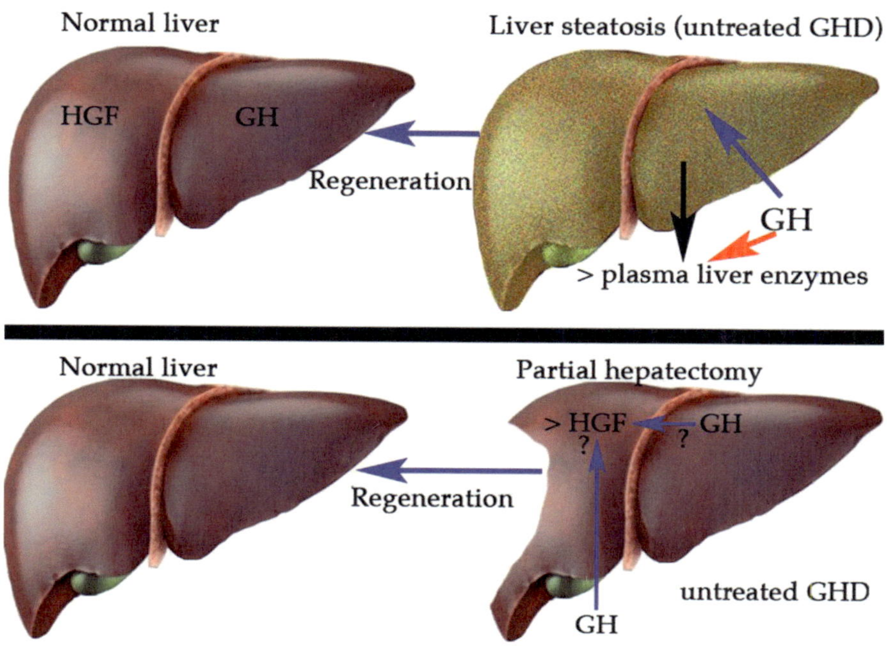

Figure 1. Effects of GH on the liver. Upper graph: There is GH expression in the normal liver (left), although this organ has its own regeneration factor (hepatocyte growth factor—HGF). Untreated GHD may suffer non-alcoholic liver steatosis (right), showing increased plasma levels of liver enzymes (transaminases); GH treatment recovers the damaged liver (blue arrows); and plasma liver enzymes come back to normal levels (red arrow). Lower graph: Untreated GHD patients cannot recover a normal liver in spite of the liver expression of GH and HGF, but GH treatment leads to regeneration of the damaged liver (blue arrows)—it is not known if this regeneration occurs because GH administration increases the hepatic expression of HGF or if it is due to a direct effect of GH on the liver.

seems to be induced by GH because hypophysectomy reduces GHR mRNA levels in rat kidneys, whereas GH therapy restores them [21]. There is also renal IGF-I biosynthesis, as it has been demonstrated in dogs [24] and confirmed by the fact that GH treatment increased IGF-I mRNA levels in the kidney of hypophysectomized rats [25, 26]. This is the reason by which GHR knockout leads to small kidneys in mice [27], and compensatory renal hypertrophy is directly dependent on GH-induced IGF-I expression [28]. It has been suggested that for GH-mediated kidney mass stimulation hepatic IGF-I production was crucial, while renal production of IGF-I has little or no effects on kidney growth [29]. In any case, studies in rodents demonstrated the importance of the GH/IGF-I system in the growth of kidneys during ontogenesis and development; however, no data indicate that a defective GH-/IGF-I signaling plays a significant role on kidney growth in humans.

In humans, short-term treatment with GH increases the glomerular filtration rate (GFR) [30]. This GH action is due to an IGF-1-mediated decrease in renal vascular resistance, leading to increased glomerular perfusion [31–33]. In addition to increasing glomerular perfusion, GH and IGF-1 augment extracellular volume and plasma volume [34], thereby also contributing to increased glomerular filtration.

The GH-IGF-1 system is a modulator of renal tubular sodium and water reabsorption [34]. Many years ago, the sodium-retaining properties of GH have been demonstrated in rats [35] and normal men [36]. This effect, traduced in an increase in extracellular volume, is stronger in men than in women [37] and seems to be dependent on the activation of the renin-angiotensin-aldosterone system because it has been seen that GH induces a rapid increase in plasma renin activity and plasma aldosterone levels in normal men [38]. However, further studies demonstrated that plasma angiotensin II and aldosterone did not increase during a treatment with GH, but plasma levels of atrial natriuretic peptide fell significantly [39]. Later studies in healthy volunteers [40] and GHD patients [41, 42] demonstrated that GH exerts a sodium-retaining effect that is independent of the renin-angiotensin-aldosterone system.

IGF-I has also antinatriuretic effects, as it has been seen in GHD children in whom the GHR is inactive because of Laron syndrome [43], and in healthy men [44]. Therefore, GH and IGF-I seem to act by different independent mechanisms in the retention of sodium by the kidney.

GH and IGF-1 are very important in the periods of increased bone formation, such as the growth stage, in which the phosphate metabolism must be well adjusted. As shown in almost 60 years ago, GH treatment led to decreased urinary phosphate excretion and increased plasma phosphate concentrations in men [45]. This effect of GH on the retention of phosphate is due to an increase in the maximum tubular phosphate reabsorption rate, as demonstrated in normal men [30] and dogs [46], and it is independent of PTH [46].

Conversely, hypophysectomy and inhibition of pulsatile GH release in rats produce increased urinary phosphorus losses [47, 48]. This has also been observed in normal humans [49–51] and in GHD patients [52–54].

As it happens with phosphate, GH and IGF-1 play an important role in adapting calcium homeostasis to the increased demands during the period of juvenile growth with accelerated bone formation. GH and IGF-1 affect calcium homeostasis mainly through their effect on vitamin D metabolism. GH stimulates calcitriol production in experimental animals [55] and men [56]; further investigations in mice and isolated cells showed that this GH action was mediated by IGF-1 stimulation of 1α-hydroxylase in the proximal tubule [57]. Chronic GH and IGF-1 deficiencies are accompanied by significant changes in renal morphology and functions, as well as by altered body composition, osteoporosis with fractures, and an increased cardiovascular risk [58–60]. Several studies have analyzed kidney size in GHD human patients. After hypophysectomy, kidney size fell by 20% after 5 months [61]. GH-untreated patients with Laron syndrome present larger ultrasonographic measured kidneys than control subjects when corrected for body surface area [62], but the kidney size is increased after long-term treatment with IGF-I [62]. GH treatment of adults with childhood-onset GH deficiency increases kidney length [63]. These effects of GH/IGF-I on the kidney are shown schematically in **Figure 2**.

The size of the kidneys in untreated GHD patients is lower than in normal people, but the administration of GH or IGF-I corrects this defect.

GH and IGF-1 deficiencies are associated with decreased glomerular filtration and renal plasma flow [64–66]. GH replacement therapy increased the GFR and renal plasma flow in some patients [64, 65] but it depends on the dose and duration of treatment. Treatment with IGF-I in patients with GH insensitivity also increases glomerular filtration [65].

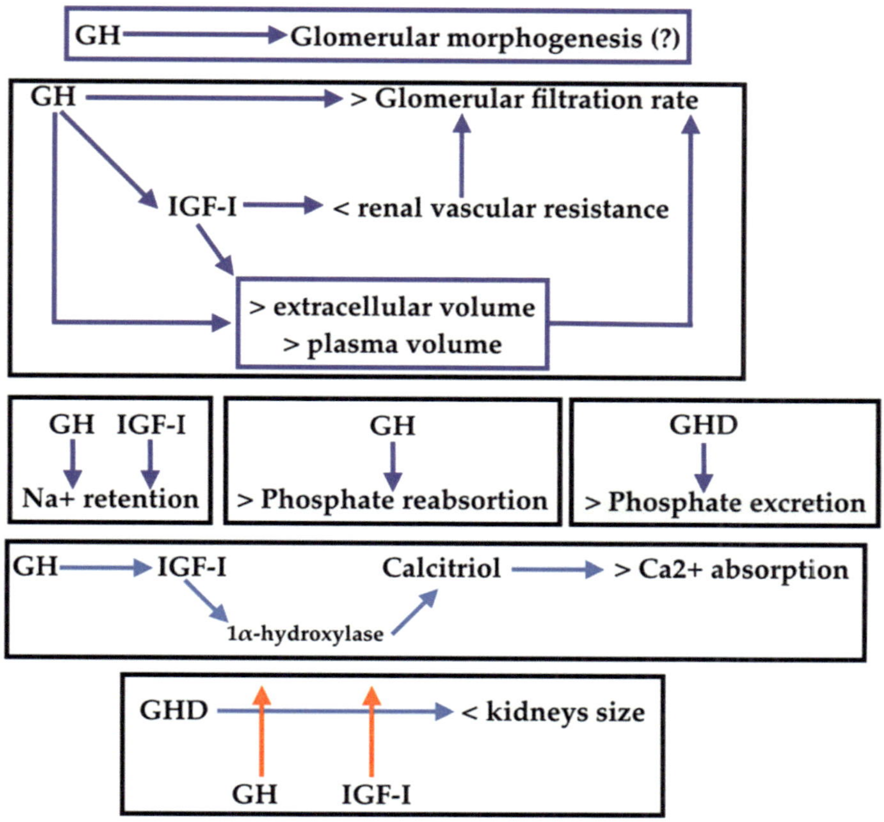

Figure 2. GH effects on the kidney. It is possible that GH participates in the early stages of the development of the kidneys by inducing glomerular morphogenesis. GH administration increases glomerular filtration rate, in this effect also participates GH-induced IGF-I, although the effects of both hormones on the glomerular filtration rate are independent. GH and IGF-I increase the retention of Na+, by decreasing its renal excretion. GH also increases the reabsorption of phosphate, while untreated GHD patients present an increase in the excretion of phosphate. GH also induces an increase in the intestinal absorption of Ca^{2+}, but this effect is mediated by IGF-I, which leads to the formation of Calcitriol.

An ancient study in hypopituitary children and young adults showed an increase in total body volume, extracellular volume, and intracellular volume after 1 year of GH therapy [67]. Two clinical trials in GHD adults posteriorly showed beneficial effects of GH treatment on body composition, with an increase in lean body mass [68, 69].

It is well known that adult GHD patients present osteoporosis with a high risk of vertebral and femoral fractures. Low bone mass can be partially improved by GH replacement [70–73] because GH therapy in GHD adults causes a transient increase in plasma calcium concentrations and urinary calcium excretion, which usually lasts between 3 and 6 months.

GH treatment increases plasma phosphate concentrations in GHD children [73, 74] and adults [52, 53, 75]. In contrast to plasma calcium concentrations, this increase in plasma phosphate persisted during 12–24 months of GH therapy [53, 73–75], while urinary phosphate excretion was decreased.

These data show the importance of GH on a normal renal function, although most of its effects at this level are mediated by IGF-I. Disordered regulation of the IGF system has been implicated in a number of kidney diseases. IGF-I activity is enhanced in early diabetic nephropathy and polycystic kidneys, whereas IGF-I resistance is found in chronic kidney failure. Moreover, IGFs have a potential role in enhancing stem cell repair after a kidney injury [76].

Importantly, children with chronic kidney disease have growth failure that can be treated with GH improving growth velocity without adverse side effects [77, 78].

For more detailed information about the effects of GH on the kidney, see [79].

1.3. GHD and adipose tissue

GH is defined as a lipolytic hormone. Untreated GHD children and adults usually present an increase in fat mass [80, 81], preferentially visceral fat; this has been attributed to the fact that GH inhibits lipid storage in adipose tissue by increasing the activity of hormone-sensitive lipase, an enzyme that plays a key role on lipolysis [82, 83], and by decreasing the inhibiting effect of insulin on hormone-sensitive lipase activity [83], although positive changes in the secretion of certain adipokines, such as adiponectin, have also been suggested as mediators of the increased adiposity in GHD states [84]. The adipose tissue is an endocrine organ that produces several hormones and cytokines that exert autocrine, paracrine, and endocrine effects. Two of these hormones, leptin and adiponectin, play very important roles in the organism. For instance, leptin is the hormone of satiety, released from adipocytes in response to food intake, and it is correlated with total fat mass. Its function, acting on its receptors in the arcuate nucleus of the hypothalamus, is related to decreasing food intake and increasing energy expenditure; conversely, adiponectin is negatively correlated with fat mass and acts as an insulin-sensitizing hormone [85]. Although it would be expected that GH effects on adipose tissue would be different in terms of leptin and adiponectin secretion, it has been seen that, in fact, these effects are negatively correlated with the release of both hormones from adipocytes. For example, in Laron syndrome, there is a marked obesity and adiponectin hypersecretion that does not change during long-term IGF-I treatment [86]. In any case, usually GH therapy reverts the increased adiposity existing in pituitary GHD children and adults [80, 81], therefore confirming the relationship between GHD and increased fat mass. Recent publications describe that in addition to its effects on the adipose tissue, GH also acts as a starvation signal that alerts the brain about energy deficiency, triggering adaptive responses to keep a minimum of energy deposits. This mechanism takes place at the central level by activating hypothalamic agouti-related protein neurons (AgRP) [87]. **Figure 3** shows how GH acts in the adipocyte.

Among other factors, since GH secretion decreases progressively from puberty, it is likely that the increase in body fat that is generally observed as we get older is related to deficient or insufficient secretion of GH. For a more detailed review of GH and the adipose tissue, see [85].

1.4. GHD and skeletal muscles

The GH-IGF-1 axis represents an important physiological mechanism to coordinate hypertrophy and postnatal skeletal muscle expansion. Both in normal rats and adult-onset GHD human patients, the administration of GH improves muscle strength and reduces body fat [88–90]. GHR-deficient mice have reduced muscle mass with defective myofiber specification and growth [91]; in skeletal muscles lacking GHR, there is a decrease in the size of myofibers, while the number of myofibers is normal. The administration of GH increases myonuclear number, facilitating the fusion of myoblasts with nascent myotubes, a mechanism mediated by the transcription factor NFATc2; however, during a time, it has been discussed if the positive actions of GH on muscle mass would be restricted to inducing enhanced uptake of amino acids by muscle, while the effects on muscle protein synthesis, and consequently the increase in muscle mass, would be dependent on GH-induced IGF-I expression, mediated by STAT5b. In fact, recent *in vitro* studies indicate that treatment of primary myoblasts with GH quickly increases IGF-I mRNA, while administration of IGF-I leads to a significant increase in primary myoblast proliferation [92]. Therefore, the role of GH on muscle would be dependent on its induction of production of IGF-I by myoblasts, and IGF-I would then be responsible for stimulating myoblasts proliferation in an autocrine manner. The real thing is that GH and IGF-I induce a hypertrophic effect on skeletal muscles by different signaling pathways, and their effects are additive (**Figure 4**). The disruption of GHR in skeletal muscle and the consequent histomorphometric changes in myofiber type and size and myonuclei number result in functionally impaired skeletal muscle. In agreement with these effects, the histology of muscles of untreated GHD patients is strongly altered, and glucose and triglyceride uptake and metabolism in skeletal muscle of GHR mutant mice are affected.

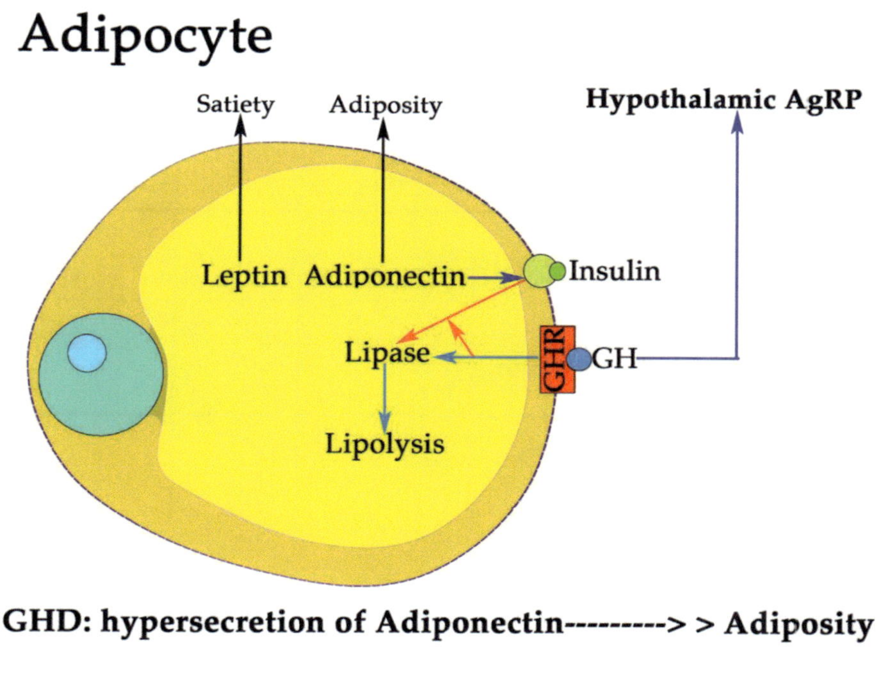

Figure 3. GH effects on fat mass. There are GHR in the membrane of adipocytes. After interacting with endocrine GH, the activity of the lipase (blue arrow) is increased leading to increased lipolysis. In addition, GH-GHR interactions lead to the inhibition of lipase activity (red arrow) induced by insulin. This insulin-inhibiting lipase activity is enhanced by adiponectin (blue arrow), a hormone secreted by adipocytes and responsible for increasing fat mass. In untreated GHD patients, there is hypersecretion of adiponectin. This is the reason by which these patients show excessive fat mass. In addition, GH acts on hypothalamic neurons that express AgRP, stimulating its production to alert the brain about energy deficiency.

In humans, a single bolus of GH induces gene expression of regulators of substrate metabolism and cellular growth of skeletal muscle *in vivo*. Some of these genes, such as *GISH* gene, seem to be directly induced by GH; however, other genes, such as *ANGPTL4* gene [93], seem to be expressed in relation to the subsequent increase in free fatty acid levels induced by GH-dependent lipolysis (**Figure 4**).

These results agree with the role that GH plays on lipid metabolism. With regard to the putative effects of GH on muscle strength, GH use has been speculated to improve physical capacity in subjects without GHD through stimulation of collagen synthesis in the tendon and skeletal muscle, which leads to better exercise training and increased muscle strength. In this context, the use of GH in healthy elderly should be an option for increasing muscle strength. However, a clinical trial showed that after 6 months of therapy, muscle strength in the bench press responsive muscles did not increase in groups treated with GH (no GHD) or placebo and showed a statistically significant increase in the leg press responsive muscles in the GH group.

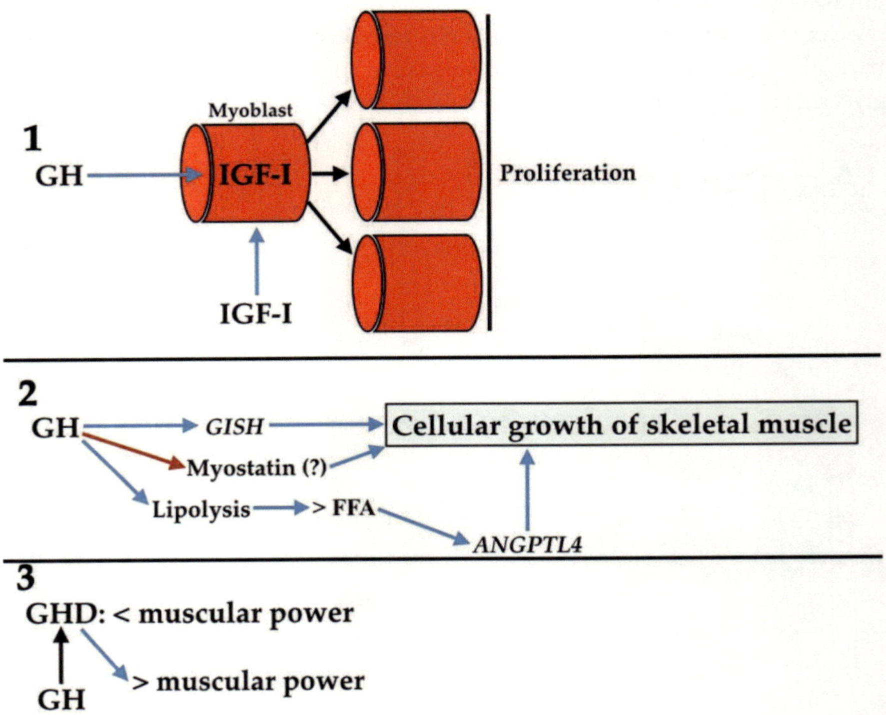

Figure 4. GH effects on skeletal muscle. 1: GH induces IGF-I expression in myoblasts. In turn, IGF-I leads to the proliferation of these myoblasts and produces muscular hypertrophy. The effects of GH and IGF-I are additive. 2: GH induces cellular growth in skeletal muscles by different mechanisms. One of them is due to the effects of GH on gene expression of regulators of substrate metabolism and cellular growth of skeletal muscle, such as *GISH*; other depends on the GH-induced lipolysis, which leads to increased levels of free fatty acids in plasma (FFA), and these stimulate the expression of *ANGPTL4* gene that acts directly on the cellular growth. In addition, GH inhibits the expression of muscular myostatin, a negative regulator of muscular growth; however, this last effect has been questioned recently. 3: According to the GH/IGF-I effects on skeletal muscles, untreated GHD patients have decreased muscular power, but this is corrected with GH treatment. Blue arrows, stimulation; red arrows, inhibition; >, increase; <, decrease.

The study demonstrated an increase in muscle strength only in the lower body part (quadriceps, for instance) after GH therapy in healthy men [94]. Therefore, GH administration does not provide significant improvements in increasing muscle power, except when GHD exists.

Of interest, sarcopenia appears while aging or after a prolonged immobilization. Although most likely this is a multifactorial process, a predominant role is played by myostatin, a muscular hormone that inhibits cell cycle progression and reduces levels of myogenic regulatory factors, thereby controlling myoblastic proliferation and differentiation during developmental myogenesis, as we and others demonstrated [95–97]. GH-induced muscular expression of the IGF-I-Akt–mTOR pathway, which mediates both differentiation in myoblasts and hypertrophy in myotubes, has been shown to inhibit myostatin-dependent signaling. Blockade of the Akt–mTOR pathway, using siRNA to RAPTOR, a component of TORC1 (TOR signaling complex 1), facilitates the inhibition by myostatin of muscle differentiation because of an increase in Smad2 phosphorylation [98]. Therefore, GH administration in these conditions of muscle wasting may be useful for recovering muscle mass at expenses of inhibiting myostatin signaling. However, a more recent study challenged these concepts, demonstrating that GH treatment in GHD did not reduce the previously elevated levels of myostatin in plasma and skeletal muscle [99]. These authors conclude that GH treatment is less effective than higher weight-based diets in increasing skeletal muscle mass. Independently of it, the role of GH/IGF-I in skeletal muscle is key and clear.

1.5. GHD and bone

The actions of the GH–IGF-I axis in the growth plate to promote longitudinal growth are already well known [100], but these are not the unique effects that the GH/IGF-I system plays at the bone level. This axis also regulates skeletal development and mineral acquisition [101]. Mouse models with disruptions of GH–IGF-I axis present a clear deterioration in parameters of bone health, dependent on GH-induced IGF-I expression, which increases bone mineral density [102]. Apart from GH, other GH-independent mechanisms regulate bone IGF-I expression, for instance, parathormone (PTH) [103]. Experimental mouse models reveal that osteoblast-derived IGF-I is a key determinant of bone mineralization. Targeted osteoblast-specific overexpression of *Igf1* via the osteocalcin promoter produced a phenotype of increased bone mineral density and trabecular bone volume [104], whereas knockout of the gene in bone (and muscle) but not liver via Cre recombinase expressed by the collagen type 1α2 promoter included a phenotype of reduced bone accretion [105].

In summary, although the effects of GH at the bone level are mainly related to the longitudinal growth of the organism before the end of puberty, and its effects are mediated by the local production of IGF-I, it cannot be discarded that GHD, both pathological and physiological (as it happens in aging), may play a role in the development of osteopenia/osteoporosis.

1.6. GHD and hematopoietic and immune systems

GH seems to play a role in the regulation of the hematopoietic system, being involved in the normal differentiation and function of blood cells [106]. GH increases plasma erythropoietin (Epo) levels and Hb in adult GHD patients [107] and increases plasma granulocyte-colony stimulating factor (G-CSF) levels and neutrophil counts in adult GHD patients [108] (**Figure 5(1)**).

Another study carried out in GHD patients treated with GH showed that the treatment significantly increased erythrocytes, Hb, and hematocrit and led to the recovery from anemia (typical of GHD patients during childhood), without affecting the number of leukocytes or platelets [109]. In all, these data indicate that GH exerts a positive role on the hematopoietic system, similar to that played by G-CSF [110]. Circulating levels of G-CSF are significantly lower in GHD than in non-GHD children, although in non-GHD children, the number of red blood cells, Hb, and hematocrit values significantly increased after 1 year of GH treatment [106]. Interestingly, unpublished data from our group indicate that short-term GH administration exerts the same effect on the hematopoietic system than G-CSF in 12-year-old Beagle dogs.

In the last years, it has been postulated that GH has a strong influence on the immune system. The production and action of immune cell-derived GH are now well known, although its important role in immunity is still being unveiled. Cells of the immune system express GH, GHRH, IGF-I, and its receptor, who through autocrine/paracrine and intracrine, but also endocrine, pathways, play a role in the immune function [111] (**Figure 5(2)**). The intracellular mechanisms of action of immune cell-derived GH are not well known, but, for instance, GH promotes the maturation and activation of dendritic cells that, as antigen-presenting cells, participate in the immune response of the organism [112].

There is GH production in lymphocytes; this GH is important for lymphocyte growth, survival, and production of cytokines [113–121]; therefore, lymphocyte GH may be an important mediator of cellular immune function mediated by the TH-1 pathway [122]. Lymphocyte GH appears to stimulate IFNγ production with a small positive effect on IL-10 production [122]. Treatment of rat lymphocytes with a specific GH antisense oligodeoxynucleotide decreased the amount of lymphocyte GH synthesized and, at the same time, reduced lymphocyte proliferation [113], what confirms the production by lymphocytes of the hormone and its effects on these cells, which is inhibited by noradrenaline and cortisol. However, it is likely that some of the effects of lymphocyte GH are due to GH-induced IGF-I production. In fact, IGF-I has also been found in lymphocytes, and studies using neutralizing antibodies to GH found that the number of cells positive for IGF-I decreased two-fold. This indicated that endogenously produced GH induces the production of IGF-I by lymphocytes [114]. Consequently, it seems that lymphocyte GH acts as an intracrine hormone [123]. It has been shown that overexpression of GH in a lymphoid cell line, devoid of the GHR, decreases the production of superoxide and increases the production of nitric oxide and the expression of IGF-I and IGF-IR, resulting in protection from apoptosis by a mechanism most likely involving an increase in the production of BcL-2 [115–118].

In all, it seems that there is a complex intracrine/autocrine regulatory circuit for the production and function of leukocyte-derived GH and IGF-I within the immune system. Therefore, this circuit could fulfill local tissue needs for these hormones independent of the pituitary or liver without disrupting homeostasis of other organ systems. For example, cells of the immune system would recognize the association of bacteria, virus, and tumors as an oxidative stress event and signal the release and transport GH, or different GH isoforms generated into the cytoplasm, and GHR into the nucleus. Once in the nucleus, GH-GHR would be free to influence transcriptional responses to the stress event and to defend the cell against oxidative damage. The results from a study by Weigent [124] support the concept that changes in the cellular redox status influence the intracellular levels of lymphocyte GH, which may exert effects on elements mediating the oxidative stress response.

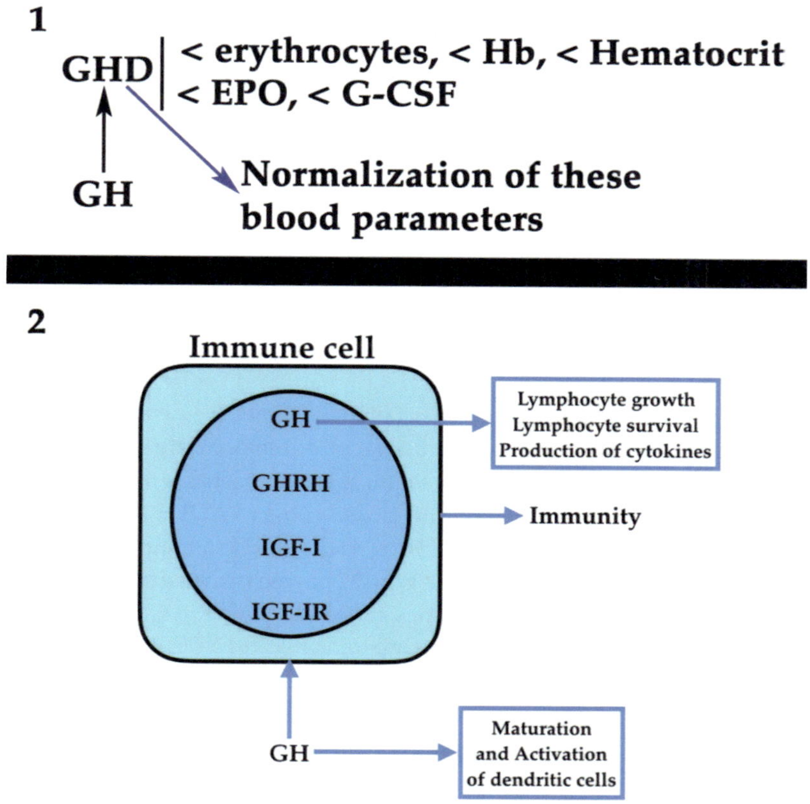

Figure 5. (1) GH plays an important role on hematopoiesis. This is the reason by which untreated GHD patients present deficits in the number of red blood cells, Hb, and hematocrit. Curiously, in these patients, there are also decreased plasma levels of EPO and G-CSF. GH administration normalizes these deficits (blue arrow) and increases plasma levels of EPO and G-CSF. (2) GH is expressed in cells of the immune system, as it happens with IGF-I and its receptor IGF-IR. There is also expression of GHRH, but its role in these immune cells is unknown. In all, these expressions contribute to increase immunity, and GH, particularly, increases the growth and survival of lymphocytes and the production of cytokines. Endocrine GH induces the activation and maturation of dendritic cells, the antigen-presenting cells. Therefore, GH and its mediators play an important role in immunity.

A very recent study indicates that GH treatment in GHD children led to some positive changes in the cellular and humoral immune profiles [125]. These data are similar to former results obtained after GH treatment in adults with childhood-onset GHD [126] and to more ancient studies in children with idiopathic short stature being treated with GH [127], although other study did not show changes in the immune function or immune parameters in GHD children after being treated with the hormone [128].

1.7. GHD and gastrointestinal functioning

Untreated GHD is associated with metabolic inflammation that usually is decreased when GH treatment is given [129]. However, situations of systemic inflammation, such as inflammatory bowel diseases (IBD), may induce GH resistance because inflammation negatively affects GH signaling. The GHR is expressed in the intestine [130, 131] for responding to GH signaling and enhancing the intestinal barrier function and mucosal healing [132, 133]. STAT5b, a key mediator of GH effects in the cells, maintains colonic barrier integrity by modulating the survival of colon epithelial cells; this is the reason by which STAT5b-deficient mice present increased susceptibility to develop colitis. In addition, GH enhances epithelial proliferation. However, the expression of GHR in the colon is reduced in patients with ulcerative colitis [134], which favors the development of resistance to the beneficial effects of GH on the function of the intestinal barrier. According to these data, it is likely that GHD patients may suffer intestinal dysfunctions. An example of it might be the relatively elevated prevalence of GHD in children suffering coeliac disease, although this disease is a genetically determined gluten-sensitive enteropathy.

1.8. GHD and adrenal glands

The system GH/IGF-I also plays a role in adrenal glands. In rats, we demonstrated that the compensatory adrenal hypertrophy that follows a unilateral adrenalectomy seems to be mediated by adrenal GH expression [135]. GH and IGF-I enhance steroidogenesis responsiveness to ACTH in cultured adrenal cells and adrenal steroid responsiveness to ACTH increases in Turner syndrome after long-term treatment with high GH doses [136]. GH is an important modulator of the activity of 11β-hydroxysteroid dehydrogenase type 1 enzyme in the adrenal gland [137], as indicated by the fact that plasma DHEAS levels are significantly lower in GHD patients (even in the patients with normal ACTH secretion) than in age-matched controls. GH replacement therapy in these GHD patients significantly increases DHEAS plasma levels. This suggests that if there is a normal secretion of ACTH, GH stimulates adrenal androgen secretion in GHD patients. Conversely, GHD patients present an increased cortisol/cortisone ratio, and GH replacement therapy reduces the increased cortisol production [138]. However, in normal subjects or laboratory animals, the stimulation of adrenal steroidogenesis by GH seems to be restricted to the fetal period [139]. Years ago, it was demonstrated that GHR is strongly expressed in the ovine fetal adrenal gland [140], but GH infusion did not affect plasma steroid levels. This suggested that the steroidogenic effects of GH may depend on the gestational age, at least in the ovine fetus.

In all, besides from the putative effects of GH on adrenal steroidogenesis, the hormone may also play a trophic regenerative role on the adrenal glands.

1.9. GHD and other effects of GH

In addition to the well-known metabolic effects of GH, and the effects of the hormone on virtually all organs and tissues of the body, reviewed previously, untreated GHD patients present some other alterations. For instance, blood pressure is higher in GHD children and adults than in normal controls [141]. This specially affects the systolic blood pressure; moreover, since GHD is associated with increased obesity, both factors contribute to increase the risk of future cardiovascular affectations. Quality of life and psychosocial behavior are affected in GHD children and adults [142], usually they are more susceptible to suffer from depression, fatigue, and less physical activity, and all these are improved after GH treatment [143]. GH is also a key modulator of neonatal hypersensitivity and pain-related behaviors during developmental inflammation. It has been found in rats in which the GHR had been deleted that there was behavioral and afferent hypersensitivity to different stimuli, mainly during early developmental stages [144].

http://dx.doi.org/10.5772/intechopen.89159

This led the authors to postulate that GH treatment might be a therapeutic weapon for pediatric pain. Regarding the effects of GH at the brain level, it has been recently shown that GHD mainly affects the brain network involving the somatosensory, somatic motor, and cerebellum networks, which may contribute to the behavioral problems existing in GHD children [145].

2. Conclusions

As it has been analyzed throughout this review, GH and its mediators play a very important role in practically the entire human organism, already from the early stages of development. This role goes far beyond than the classical concepts attributing to the hormone a merely metabolic role and an effect on longitudinal growth. Besides the pituitary production of GH that acts as an endocrine hormone, there is a peripheral production of GH that acts in autocrine/paracrine and even intracrine in the cells, which produce it. As a consequence of its physiological actions, the deficit of GH or its receptor leads to very important affectations. Consequently, GH replacement therapy improves the affectations occurring in GHD patients and their quality of life. Since GH secretion declines progressively from 20 years of age until being practically undetectable from 50 years old, it is likely that most of the age-related diseases and the decreased quality of life occur as a consequence of the absence of this hormone. In some cases, GH acts coordinately with other hormones; therefore, for carrying out some of its effects, it has to be considered as a co-hormone.

Acknowledgements

We thank the therapists of Foltra Medical Center (Teo, Spain) and researchers from the Department of Physiology of the Faculty of Medicine of the University of Santiago de Compostela who contributed their work to a large part of the information provided in this review. We also acknowledge the Foltra Foundation (Teo, Spain) for the help provided to write this review. This review has been funded by Foundation Foltra (Teo, Spain), grant F2019-7.

Conflict of interest

The author declares that there is not any conflict of interest.

Author details

Jesús Devesa

Address all correspondence to: devesa.jesus@gmail.com

Scientific Direction, Medical Center Foltra, Teo, Spain

References

[1] Cui Y, Hosui A, Sun R, Shen K, Gavrilova O, Chen W, et al. Loss of signal transducer and activator of transcription 5 leads to hepatosteatosis and impaired liver regeneration. Hepatology. 2007;**46**:504-513. DOI: 10.1002/hep.21713

[2] Fan Y, Menon RK, Cohen P, Hwang D, Clemens T, DiGirolamo DJ, et al. Liver-specific deletion of the growth hormone receptor reveals essential role of growth hormone signaling in hepatic lipid metabolism. The Journal of Biological Chemistry. 2009;**284**:19937-19944. DOI: 10.1074/jbc.MC109.014308

[3] Sos BC, Harris C, Nordstrom SM, Tran JL, Balázs M, Caplazi P, et al. Abrogation of growth hormone secretion rescues fatty liver in mice with hepatocyte-specific deletion of JAK2. The Journal of Clinical Investigation. 2011;**121**:1412-1423. DOI: 10.1172/JCI42894

[4] Nishizawa H, Iguchi G, Murawaki A, Fukuoka H, Hayashi Y, Kaji H, et al. Nonalcoholic fatty liver disease in adult hypopituitary patients with GH deficiency and the impact of GH replacement therapy. European Journal of Endocrinology. 2012;**167**:67-74. DOI: 10.1530/EJE-12-0252

[5] Takahashi Y, Iida K, Takahashi K, Yoshioka S, Fukuoka H, Takeno R, et al. Growth hormone reverses nonalcoholic steatohepatitis in a patient with adult growth hormone deficiency. Gastroenterology. 2007;**132**:938-943. DOI: 10.1053/j.gastro.2006.12.024

[6] Xu L, Xu C, Yu C, Miao M, Zhang X, Zhu Z, et al. Association between serum growth hormone levels and nonalcoholic fatty liver disease: A cross-sectional study. PLoS One. 2012;**7**:e44136. DOI: 10.1371/journal.pone.0044136

[7] Matsumoto R, Fukuoka H, Iguchi G, Nishizawa H, Bando H, Suda K, et al. Long-term effects of growth hormone replacement therapy on liver function in adult patients with growth hormone deficiency. Growth Hormone & IGF Research. 2014;**24**:174-179. DOI: 10.1016/j.ghir.2014.07.002

[8] Takano S, Kanzaki S, Sato M, Kubo T, Seino Y. Effect of growth hormone on fatty liver in panhypopituitarism. Archives of Disease in Childhood. 1997;**76**:537-538. DOI: 10.1136/adc.76.6.537

[9] Gilliland T, Dufour S, Shulman GI, Petersen KF, Emre SH. Resolution of non-alcoholic steatohepatitis after growth hormone replacement in a pediatric liver transplant patient with panhypopituitarism. Pediatric Transplantation. 2016;**20**:1157-1163. DOI: 10.1111/petr.12819

[10] Wada K, Kobayashi H, Moriyama A, Haneda Y, Mushimoto Y, Hasegawa Y, et al. A case of an infant with congenital combined pituitary hormone deficiency and normalized liver histology of infantile chole- stasis after hormone replacement therapy. Clinical Pediatric Endocrinology. 2017;**26**:251-257. DOI: 10.1297/cpe.26.251

[11] Rufinatscha K, Ress C, Folie S, Haas S, Salzmann K, Moser P, et al. Metabolic effects of reduced growth hormone action in fatty liver disease. Hepatology International. 2018;**12**:474-481. DOI: 10.1007/s12072-018-9893-7

[12] Miranda-Lora AL, Zamora-Nava LE, Marín-Rosas DL, Klünder-Klünder M, Sánchez-Curiel M, Dies-Suárez P. Resolution of fatty liver disease after growth hormone replacement in a pediatric survivor of thyroid cancer. Boletín Médico del Hospital Infantil de México. 2019;**76**:38-145. DOI: 10.24875/BMHIM.18000114

[13] Nakamura T, Nawa K, Ichihara A. Partial purification and characterization of hepatocyte growth factor from serum of hepatectomized rats. Biochemical and Biophysical Research Communications. 1984;**122**:1450-1459. DOI: 10.1016/0006-291x(84)91253-1

[14] Nakamura T. Structure and function of hepatocyte growth factor. Progress in Growth Factor Research. 1991;**3**:67-85. DOI: 10.1016/0955-2235(91)90014-U

[15] Kinoshita T, Hirao S, Matsumoto K, Nakamura T. Possible endocrine control by hepatocyte growth factor of liver regeneration after partial hepatectomy. Biochemical and Biophysical Research Communications. 1991;**17**:330-335. DOI: 10.1016/0006-291x(91)91987-n

[16] Matsumoto K, Nakamura T. Hepatocyte growth factor: Molecular structure, roles in liver regeneration, and other biological functions. Critical Reviews in Oncogenesis. 1992;**3**:27-54. DOI: 10.1111/j.1440-1746.1991.tb00897.x

[17] Birchmeier C, Gherardi E. Developmental roles of HGF/SF and its receptor, the c-met tyrosine kinase. Trends in Cell Biology. 1998;**8**:404-410. DOI: 10.1016/S0962-8924(98)01359-2

[18] Fausto N, Campbell JS, Riehle KJ. Liver regeneration. Hepatology. 2006;**43**(Suppl 1):S45-S53. DOI: 10.1002/hep.20969

[19] Ekberg S, Luther M, Nakamura T, Jansson JO. Growth hormone promotes early initiation of hepatocyte growth factor gene expression in the liver of hypophysectomized rats after partial hepatectomy. The Journal of Endocrinology. 1992;**135**:59-67. DOI: 10.1677/joe.0.1350059

[20] Devesa J, Almengló C, Devesa P. Multiple effects of growth hormone in the body: Is it really the hormone for growth? Clinical Medicine Insights: Endocrinology and Diabetes. 2016;**9**:47-71. DOI: 10.4137(CMED.S38201

[21] Chin E, Zhou J, Bondy CA. Renal growth hormone receptor gene expression: Relationship to renal insulin-like growth factor system. Endocrinology. 1992;**131**:3061-3066. DOI: 10.1210/endo.131.6.1446640

[22] Lobie PE, García-Aragón J, Wang BS, Baumbach WR, Waters MJ. Cellular localization of the growth hormone binding protein in the rat. Endocrinology. 1992;**130**:3057-3065. DOI: 10.1210/endo.130.5.1374020

[23] Simard M, Manthos H, Giaid A, Lefèbvre Y, Goodyer CG. Ontogeny of growth hormone receptors in human tissues: An immunohistochemical study. The Journal of Clinical Endocrinology and Metabolism. 1996;**81**:3097-3102. DOI: 10.1210/jcem.81.8.8768881

[24] Schimpff RM, Donnadieu M, Duval M. Serum somatomedin activity measured as sulphation factor in peripheral, hepatic and renal veins in normal mongrel dogs: Early effects of intravenous injection of growth hormone. Acta Endocrinologica. 1980;**93**:155-161. DOI: 10.1530/acta.0.0930155

[25] Murphy LJ, Bell GI, Friesen HG. Growth hormone stimulates sequential induction of c-myc and insulin-like growth factor I expression in vivo. Endocrinology. 1987;**120**:1806-1812. DOI: 10.1210/endo-120-5-1806

[26] Roberts CT Jr, Lasky SR, Lowe WL Jr, Seaman WT, LeRoith D. Molecular cloning of rat insulin-like growth factor I complementary deoxyribonucleic acids: Differential messenger ribonucleic acid processing and regulation by growth hormone in extrahepatic tissues. Molecular Endocrinology. 1987;**1**:243-248. DOI: 10.1210/mend-1-3-243

[27] List EO, Sackmann-Sala L, Berryman DE, Funk K, Kelder B, Gosney ES, et al. Endocrine parameters and phenotypes of the growth hormone receptor gene disrupted (GHR−/−) mouse. Endocrine Reviews. 2011;**32**:356-386. DOI: 10.1210/er.2010-0009

[28] Flyvbjerg A, Bennett WF, Rasch R, van Neck JW, Groffen CA, Kopchick JJ, et al. Compensatory renal growth in uninephrectomized adult mice is growth hormone dependent. Kidney International. 1999;**56**:2048-2054. DOI: 10.1046/j.1523-1755.1999.00776.x

[29] Nordstrom SM, Tran JL, Sos BC, Wagner KU, Weiss EJ. Liver-derived IGF-I contributes to GH-dependent increases in lean mass and bone mineral density in mice with comparable levels of circulating GH. Molecular Endocrinology. 2011;**25**:1223-1230. DOI: 10.1210/me.2011-0047

[30] Corvilain J, Abramow M, Bergans A. Some effects of human growth hormone on renal hemodynamics and on tubular posphate transport in man. The Journal of Clinical Investigation. 1962;**41**:1230-1235. DOI: 10.1172/JCI104584

[31] Guler HP, Schmid C, Zapf J, Froesch ER. Effects of recombinant insulin-like growth factor I on insulin secretion and renal function in normal human subjects. Proceedings of the National Academy of Sciences of the United States of America. 1989;**86**:2868-2872. DOI: 10.1073/pnas.86.8.2868

[32] Hirschberg R, Rabb H, Bergamo R, Kopple JD. The delayed effect of growth hormone on renal function in humans. Kidney International. 1989;**35**:865-870. DOI: 10.1038/ki.1989.65

[33] Guler HP, Eckardt KU, Zapf J, Bauer C, Froesch ER. Insulin-like growth factor I increase glomerular filtration rate and renal plasma flow in man. European Journal of Endocrinology. 1989;**121**:101-106. DOI: 10.1530/acta.0.1210101

[34] Møller J. Effects of growth hormone on fluid homeostasis. Clinical and experimental aspects. Growth Hormone & IGF Research. 2003;**13**:55-74. DOI: 10.1016/S1096-6374(03)00011-X

[35] Whitney JE, Bennett LL, Li CH. Reduction of urinary sodium and potassium produced by growth hormone in normal female rats. Proceedings of the Society for Experimental Biology and Medicine. 1952;**79**:584-587. DOI: 10.3181/00379727-79-19454

[36] Beck JC, McGarry EE, Dyrenfurth I, Venning EH. Metabolic effects of human and monkey growth hormone in man. Science. 1957;**125**:884-105. DOI: 10.1126/science.125.3253.884

[37] Ehrnborg C, Ellegård L, Bosaeus I, Bengtsson BA, Rosén T. Supraphysiological growth hormone: Less fat, more extracellular fluid but uncertain effects on muscles in healthy, active young adults. Clinical Endocrinology. 2005;**62**:449-457. DOI: 10.1111/j.1365-2265.2005.02240.x

[38] Ho KY, Weissberger AJ. The antinatriuretic action of biosynthetic human growth hormone in man involves activation of the renin-angiotensin system. Metabolism. 1990;**39**:133-137. DOI: 10.1016/0026-0495(90)90065-K

[39] Møller J, Jørgensen JO, Møller N, Hansen KW, Pedersen EB, Christiansen JS. Expansion of extracellular volume and suppression of atrial natriuretic peptide after growth hormone administration in normal man. The Journal of Clinical Endocrinology and Metabolism. 1991;**72**:768-772. DOI: 10.1210/jcem-72-4-768

[40] Hansen TK, Møller J, Thomsen K, Frandsen E, Dall R, Jørgensen JO, et al. Effects of growth hormone on renal tubular handling of sodium in healthy humans. American Journal of Physiology. Endocrinology and Metabolism. 2001;**281**:E1326-E1332. DOI: 10.1152/ajpendo.2001.281.6.E1326

[41] Johannsson G, Sverrisdóttir YB, Ellegård L, Lundberg PA, Herlitz H. GH increases extracellular volume by stimulating sodium reabsorption in the distal nephron and preventing pressure natriuresis. The Journal of Clinical Endocrinology and Metabolism. 2002;**87**:1743-1749. DOI: 10.1210/jcem.87.4.8394

[42] Johannsson G, Gibney J, Wolthers T, Leung KC, Ho KK. Independent and combined effects of testosterone and growth hormone on extracellular water in hypopituitary men. The Journal of Clinical Endocrinology and Metabolism. 2005;**90**:3989-3994. DOI: 10.1210/jc.2005-0553

[43] Walker JL, Ginalska-Malinowska M, Romer TE, Pucilowska JB, Underwood LE. Effects of the infusion of insulin-like growth factor I in a child with growth hormone insensitivity syndrome (Laron dwarfism). The New England Journal of Medicine. 1991;**324**:1483-1488. DOI: 10.1056/NEJM199105233242107

[44] Møller J, Jørgensen JO, Marqversen J, Frandsen E, Christiansen JS. Insulin-like growth factor I administration induces fluid and sodium retention in healthy adults: Possible involvement of renin and atrial natriuretic factor. Clinical Endocrinology. 2000;**52**:181-186. DOI: 10.1046/j.1365-2265.2000.00931.x

[45] Henneman PH, Forbes AP, Moldawer M, Dempsey EF, Carroll EL. Effects of human growth hormone in man. The Journal of Clinical Investigation. 1960;**39**:1223-1238. DOI: 10.1172/JCI104138

[46] Corvilain J, Abramow M. Effect of growth hormone on tubular transport of phosphate in normal and parathyroidectomized dogs. The Journal of Clinical Investigation. 1964;**43**:1608-1612. DOI: 10.1172/JCI105036

[47] Caverzasio J, Faundez R, Fleisch H, Bonjour JP. Tubular adaptation to pi restriction in hypophysectomized rats. Pflügers Archiv. 1981;**392**:17-21. DOI: 10.1007/BF00584576

[48] Mulroney SE, Lumpkin MD, Haramati A. Suppression of growth hormone release restores phosphaturic response to PTH in immature rats. The American Journal of Physiology. 1991;**261**(6 Pt 2):F1110-F1113. DOI: 10.1152/ajprenal.1991.261.6.F1110

[49] Marcus R, Butterfield G, Holloway L, Gilliland L, Baylink DJ, Hintz RL, et al. Effects of short-term administration of recombinant human growth hormone to elderly people. The Journal of Clinical Endocrinology and Metabolism. 1990;**70**:519-527. DOI: 10.1210/jcem-70-2-519

[50] Holloway L, Butterfield G, Hintz RL, Gesundheit N, Marcus R. Effects of recombinant human growth hormone on metabolic indices, body composition, and bone turnover

in healthy elderly women. The Journal of Clinical Endocrinology and Metabolism. 1994;**79**:470-479. DOI: 10.1210/jcem.79.2.7519191

[51] Joseph F, Ahmad AM, Ul-Haq M, Durham BH, Whittingham P, Fraser WD, et al. Effects of growth hormone administration on bone mineral metabolism, PTH sensitivity and PTH secretory rhythm in postmenopausal women with established osteoporosis. Journal of Bone and Mineral Research. 2008;**23**:721-729. DOI: 10.1359/jbmr.071117

[52] Bengtsson BA, Edén S, Lönn L, Kvist H, Stokland A, Lindstedt G, et al. Treatment of adults with growth hormone (GH) deficiency with recombinant human GH. The Journal of Clinical Endocrinology and Metabolism. 1993;**76**:309-317. DOI: 10.1210/jcem.76.2.8432773

[53] Ahmad AM, Thomas J, Clewes A, Hopkins MT, Guzder R, Ibrahim H, et al. Effects of growth hormone replacement on parathyroid hormone sensitivity and bone mineral metabolism. The Journal of Clinical Endocrinology and Metabolism. 2003;**88**:2860-2868. DOI: 10.1210/jc.2002-021787

[54] White HD, Ahmad AM, Durham BH, Patwala A, Whittingham P, Fraser WD, et al. Growth hormone replacement is important for the restoration of parathyroid hormone sensitivity and improvement in bone metabolism in older adult growth hormone-deficient patients. The Journal of Clinical Endocrinology and Metabolism. 2005;**90**:3371-3380. DOI: 10.1210/jc.2004-1650

[55] Spanos E, Barrett D, MacIntyre I, Pike JW, Safilian EF, Haussler MR. Effect of growth hormone on vitamin D metabolism. Nature. 1978;**273**:246-247. DOI: 10.1038/273246a0

[56] Brown DJ, Spanos E, MacIntyre I. Role of pituitary hormones in regulating renal vitamin D metabolism in man. British Medical Journal. 1980;**280**:277-278. DOI: 10.1136/bmj.280.6210.277

[57] Menaa C, Vrtovsnik F, Friedlander G, Corvol M, Garabédian M. Insulin-like growth factor I, a unique calcium-dependent stimulator of 1,25-dihydroxyvitamin D3 production. Studies in cultured mouse kidney cells. The Journal of Biological Chemistry. 1995;**270**:25461-25467. DOI: 10.1074/jbc.270.43.25461

[58] Gola M, Bonadonna S, Doga M, Giustina A. Clinical review: Growth hormone and cardiovascular risk factors. The Journal of Clinical Endocrinology and Metabolism. 2005;**90**:1864-1870. DOI: 10.1210/jc.2004-0545

[59] Mazziotti G, Bianchi A, Bonadonna S, Nuzzo M, Cimino V, Fusco A, et al. Increased prevalence of radiological spinal deformities in adult patients with GH deficiency: Influence of GH replacement therapy. Journal of Bone and Mineral Research. 2006;**21**. DOI: 520:8. DOI: 10.1359/JBMR.050603

[60] Maison P, Griffin S, Nicoue-Beglah M, Haddad N, Balkau B, Chanson P. Impact of growth hormone (GH) treatment on cardiovascular risk factors in GH-deficient adults: A Metaanalysis of blinded, randomized, placebo-controlled trials. The Journal of Clinical Endocrinology and Metabolism. 2004;**89**:2192-2199. DOI: 10.1210/jc.2003-030840

[61] Falkhedent T, Sjoegren B. Extracellular fluid volume and renal function in pituitary insufficiency and acromegaly. Acta Endocrinologica. 1964;**46**:80-8l. DOI: 10.1530/acta.0.0460080

[62] Oliveira CR, Salvatori R, Nóbrega LM, Carvalho EO, Menezes M, Farias CT, et al. Sizes of abdominal organs in adults with severe short stature due to severe, untreated, congenital GH deficiency caused by a homozygous mutation in the GHRH receptor gene. Clinical Endocrinology. 2008;**69**:153-158. DOI: 10.1111/j.1365-2265.2007.03148.x

[63] Link K, Bülow B, Westman K, Salmonsson EC, Eskilsson J, Erfurth EM. Low individualized growth hormone (GH) dose increased renal and cardiac growth in young adults with childhood onset GH deficiency. Clinical Endocrinology. 2001;**55**:741-748. DOI: 10.1046/j.1365-2265.2001.01413.x

[64] Jørgensen JO, Pedersen SA, Thuesen L, Jørgensen J, Ingemann-Hansen T, Skakkebaek NE, et al. Beneficial effects of growth hormone treatment in GH-deficient adults. Lancet. 1989;**1**:1221-1225. DOI: 10.1016/s0140-6736(89)92328-3

[65] Caidahl K, Edén S, Bengtsson BA. Cardiovascular and renal effects of growth hormone. Clinical Endocrinology. 1994;**40**:393-400. DOI: 10.1111/j.1365-2265.1994.tb03937.x

[66] Klinger B, Laron Z. Renal function in Laron syndrome patients treated by insulin-like growth factor-I. Pediatric Nephrology. 1994 Dec;**8**(6):684-688. DOI: 10.1007/BF00869089

[67] Parra A, Argote RM, García G, Cervantes C, Alatorre S, Pérez-Pasten E. Body composition in hypopituitary dwarfs before and during human growth hormone therapy. Metabolism. 1979;**28**:851-857. DOI: 10.1016/0026-0495(79)90212-9

[68] Whitehead HM, Boreham C, McIlrath EM, Sheridan B, Kennedy L, Atkinson AB, et al. Growth hormone treatment of adults with growth hormone deficiency: Results of a 13-month placebo controlled cross-over study. Clinical Endocrinology. 1992;**36**:45-52. DOI: 10.1111/j.1365-2265.1992.tb02901.x

[69] Binnerts A, Deurenberg P, Swart GR, Wilson JH, Lamberts SW. Body composition in growth hormone-deficient adults. The American Journal of Clinical Nutrition. 1992;**55**:918-923. DOI: 10.1093/ajcn/55.5.918

[70] Kaufman JM, Taelman P, Vermeulen A, Vandeweghe M. Bone mineral status in growth hormone-deficient males with isolated and multiple pituitary deficiencies of childhood onset. The Journal of Clinical Endocrinology and Metabolism. 1992;**74**:118-123. DOI: 10.1210/jcem.74.1.1727808

[71] O'Halloran DJ, Tsatsoulis A, Whitehouse RW, Holmes SJ, Adams JE, Shalet SM. Increased bone density after recombinant human growth hormone (GH) therapy in adults with isolated GH deficiency. The Journal of Clinical Endocrinology and Metabolism. 1993;**76**:1344-1348

[72] Holmes SJ, Economou G, Whitehouse RW, Adams JE, Shalet SM. Reduced bone mineral density in patients with adult onset growth hormone deficiency. The Journal of Clinical Endocrinology and Metabolism. 1994;**78**:669-674. DOI: 10.1210/jcem.78.3.8126140

[73] Boot AM, Engels MA, Boerma GJ, Krenning EP, De Muinck Keizer-Schrama SM. Changes in bone mineral density, body composition, and lipid metabolism during growth hormone (GH) treatment in children with GH deficiency. The Journal of Clinical Endocrinology and Metabolism. 1997;**82**:2423-2428. DOI: 10.1210/jcem.82.8.4149

[74] Saggese G, Baroncelli GI, Bertelloni S, Cinquanta L, Di Nero G. Effects of long-term treatment with growth hormone on bone and mineral metabolism in children with growth hormone deficiency. The Journal of Pediatrics. 1993;**122**:37-45. DOI: 10.1016//S0022-3476(05)83484-5

[75] Hansen TB, Brixen K, Vahl N, Jørgensen JO, Christiansen JS, Mosekilde L, et al. Effects of 12 months of growth hormone (GH) treatment on calciotropic hormones, calcium homeostasis, and bone metabolism in adults with acquired GH deficiency: A double blind, randomized, placebo-controlled study. The Journal of Clinical Endocrinology and Metabolism. 1996;**81**:3352-3359. DOI: 10.1210/jcem.81.9.8784096

[76] Bach LA, Hale LJ. Insulin-like growth factors and kidney disease. American Journal of Kidney Diseases. 2015;**65**:327-336. DOI: 10.1053/j.ajkd/2014.05.024

[77] Müller-Wiefel D, Frisch H, Tulassay T, Bell L, Zadik Z. Treatment of growth failure with growth hormone in children with chronic kidney disease: An open-label long-term study. Clinical Nephrology. 2010;**74**:97-105. DOI: 10.5414/cnp74097

[78] Mehls O, Lindberg A, Haffner D, Schaefer F, Wühl E. Long-term treatment growth hormone treatment in short children with CKD does not accelerate decline of renal function: Results from the KIGS registry and ESCAPE trial. Pediatric Nephrology. 2015;**30**:2145-2151. DOI: 10.1007/s00467-015-3157-8

[79] Kamenicky P, Mazziotti G, Lombès M, Giustina A, Chanson P. Growth hormone, insulin-like growth factor-1, and the kidney: Pathophysiological and clinical implications. Endocrine Reviews. 2014;**35**:234-281. DOI: 10.1210/er.2013-1071

[80] Beshyah SA, Freemantle C, Thomas E, et al. Abnormal body composition and reduced bone mass in growth hormone deficient hypopituitary adults. Clinical Endocrinology. 1995;**42**:179-189. DOI: 10.1111/j.1365-2265.1995.tb01860.x

[81] Møller N, Jørgensen JO. Effects of growth hormone on glucose, lipid, and protein metabolism in human subjects. Endocrine Reviews. 2009;**30**:152-177. DOI: 10.1210/er.2008-0027

[82] Dietz J, Schwartz J. Growth hormone alters lipolysis and hormone-sensitive lipase activity in 3T3-F442A adipocytes. Metabolism. 1991;**40**:800-806. DOI: 10.1016/0026-0495(91)90006-I

[83] Johansen T, Richelsen B, Hansen HS, Din N, Malmlöf K. Growth hormone- mediated breakdown of body fat: Effects of GH on lipases in adipose tissue and skeletal muscle of old rats fed different diets. Hormone and Metabolic Research. 2003;**35**:243-250. DOI: 10.1055/s-2003-39481

[84] List EO, Berryman DE, Funk K, Gosney ES, Jara A, Kelder B, et al. The role of GH in adipose tissue: Lessons from adipose-specific GH receptor gene-disrupted mice. Molecular Endocrinology. 2013;**27**:524-535. DOI: 10.1210/me.2012-1330

[85] Berryman DE, List EO. Growth hormone's effect on adipose tissue: Quality versus quantity. International Journal of Molecular Sciences. 2017;**18**:1621. DOI: 10.3390/ijms18081621

[86] Kanety H, Hemi R, Ginsberg S, Pariente C, Yissachar E, Barhod E, et al. Total and high molecular weight adiponectin are elevated in patients with Laron syndrome despite marked obesity. European Journal of Endocrinology. 2009;**161**:837-844. DOI: 10.1530/EJE-09-0419

[87] Furigo IC, Teixeira PDS, de Souza GO, Couto GCL, Romero GG, Perelló M, et al. Growth hormone regulates neuroendocrine responses to weight loss via AgRP neurons. Nature Communications. 2019;**10**:662. DOI: 10.1038/s41467-019-08607-1

[88] Ullman M, Oldfors A. Effects of growth hormone on skeletal muscle I. Studies on normal adult rats. Acta Physiologica Scandinavica. 1989;**135**:531-536. DOI: 10.1111/j.1748-1716.1989.tb08612.x

[89] Baum HB, Biller BM, Finkelstein JS, Cannistraro KB, Oppenheim DS, Schoenfeld DA, et al. Effects of physiologic growth hormone therapy on bone density and body composition in patients with adult-onset growth hormone deficiency. A randomized, placebo-controlled trial. Annals of Internal Medicine. 1996;**125**:883-890. DOI: 10.7326/0003-4819-125-11-199612010-00003

[90] Weber MM. Effects of growth hormone on skeletal muscle. Hormone Research. 2002;**58**(Suppl 3):43-48. DOI: 10.1159/000066482

[91] Sotiropoulos A, Ohanna M, Kedzia C, Menon RK, Kopchik JJ, Kelly PA, et al. Growth hormone promotes skeletal muscle cell fusion independent of insulin-like growth factor 1 up-regulation. Proceedings of the National Academy of Sciences of the United States of America. 2006;**103**:7315-7320. DOI: 10.1073/pnas.0510033103

[92] Mavalli MD, DiGirolamo DJ, Fan Y, Riddle RC, Campbell KS, van Groen T, et al. Distinct growth hormone receptor signaling modes regulate skeletal muscle development and insulin sensitivity in mice. The Journal of Clinical Investigation. 2010;**120**:4007-4020. DOI: 10.1172/JCI42447

[93] Clasen BF, Krusenstjerna-Hafstrøm T, Holm Vendelbo MH, Thorsen K, Escande C, Møller N, et al. Gene expression in skeletal muscle after an acute intravenous GH bolus in human subjects: Identification of a mechanism regulating ANGPTL4. Journal of Lipid Research. 2013;**54**:1988-1997. DOI: 10.1194/jlr.P034520

[94] Tavares AB, Micmacher E, Biesek S, et al. Effects of growth hormone administration on muscle strength in men over 50 years old. International Journal of Endocrinology. 2013;**2013**:942030-942036. DOI: 10.1155/2013/942030

[95] Thomas M, Langley B, Berry C, Sharma M, Kirk S, Bass J, et al. Myostatin, a negative regulator of muscle growth, functions by inhibiting myoblast proliferation. The Journal of Biological Chemistry. 2000;**275**:40235-40243. DOI: 10.1074/jbc.M004356200

[96] Ríos R, Carneiro I, Arce VM, Devesa J. Myostatin is an inhibitor of myogenic differentiation. American Journal of Physiology. Cell Physiology. 2002;**282**:C993-C999. DOI: 10.1152/ajpcell.00372.2001

[97] Langley B, Thomas M, Bishop A, Sharma M, Gilmour S, Kambadur R. Myostatin inhibits myoblast differentiation by down-regulating MyoD expression. The Journal of Biological Chemistry. 2002;**277**:49831-49840. DOI: 10.1074/jbc.M204291200

[98] Trendelenburg AU, Meyer A, Rohner D, Boyle J, Hatakeyama S, Glass DJ. Myostatin reduces Akt/TORC1/p70S6K signaling, inhibiting myoblast differentiation and myotube size. American Journal of Physiology. Cell Physiology. 2009;**296**:C1258-C1270. DOI: 10.1152/ajpcell.00105.2009

[99] Paul RG, McMahon CD, Elston MS, Conaglen JV. GH replacement titrated to serum IGF-1 does not reduce concentrations of myostatin in blood or skeletal muscle. Growth Hormone & IGF Research. 2019;**44**:11-16. DOI: 10.1016/j.ghir.2018.12.001

[100] Nilsson O, Marino R, De Luca F, Philip M, Baron J. Endocrine regulation of the growth plate. Hormone Research. 2005;**64**:157-165. DOI: 10.1159/000088791

[101] Yakar S, Courtland HW, Clemmons D. IGF-1 and bone: New discoveries from mouse models. Journal of Bone and Mineral Research. 2010;**25**:2543-2552. DOI: 10.1002/jbmr.234

[102] Yakar S, Rosen CJ, Beamer WG, Ackert-Bicknell CL, Wu Y, Liu JL, et al. Circulating levels of IGF-1 directly regulate bone growth and density. The Journal of Clinical Investigation. 2002;**110**:771-781. DOI: 10.1172/JCI15463

[103] Bikle DD, Sakata T, Leary C, Elalieh H, Ginziger D, Rosen CJ, et al. Insulin-like growth factor I is required for the anabolic actions of parathyroid hormone on mouse bone. Journal of Bone and Mineral Research. 2002;**17**:1570-1578. DOI: 10.1359/jbmr.2002.17.9.1570

[104] Zhao G, Monier-Faugere MC, Langub MC, Geng Z, Nakayama T, Pike JW, et al. Targeted overexpression of insulin-like growth factor I to osteoblasts of transgenic mice: Increased trabecular bone volume without increased osteoblast proliferation. Endocrinology. 2000;**141**:2674-2682. DOI: 10.1210/endo.141.7.7585

[105] Govoni KE, Wergedal JE, Florin L, Angel P, Baylink DJ, Mohan S. Conditional deletion of insulin-like growth factor-I in collagen type 1α2-expressing cells results in postnatal lethality and a dramatic reduction in bone accretion. Endocrinology. 2007;**148**:5706-5715. DOI: 10.1210/en.2007-0608

[106] Meazza C, Bonomelli I, Pagani S, Travaglino P, Laarej K, Cantoni F, et al. Effect of human recombinant growth hormone therapy on circulating levels of erythropoietin and granulocyte-colony stimulating factor in short children. Journal of Pediatric Endocrinology & Metabolism. 2009;**22**:837-843. DOI: 10.1515/JPEM.2009.22.9.837

[107] Sohmiya M, Kato Y. Effect of long-term administration of recombinant human growth hormone (rhGH) on plasma erythropoietin (EPO) and haemoglobin levels in anaemic patients with adult GH deficiency. Clinical Endocrinology. 2001;**55**:749-754. DOI: 10.1046/j.1365-2265.2001.01417.x

[108] Sohmiya M, Kanazawa I, Kato Y. Effect of recombinant human GH on circulating granulocyte colony-stimulating factor and neutrophils in patients with adult GH deficiency. European Journal of Endocrinology. 2005;**152**:211-215. DOI: 10.1530/eje.1.01831

[109] Esposito A, Capalbo D, De Martino L, et al. Long-term effects of growth hormone (GH) replacement therapy on hematopoiesis in a large cohort of children with GH deficiency. Endocrine. 2016;**53**:192-198. DOI: 10.1007/s12020-015-0781-9

[110] Carlo-Stella C, Di Nicola M, Milani R, Longoni P, Milanesi M, Bifulco C, et al. Age- and irradiation-associated loss of bone marrow hematopoietic function in mice is reversed by recombinant human growth hormone. Experimental Hematology. 2004;**32**:171-178. DOI: 10.1016/j.exphem.2003.11.007

[111] Weigent DA. Lymphocyte GH-axis hormones in immunity. Cellular Immunology. 2013;**285**:118-132. DOI: 10.1016/j.cellimm.2013.10.003

[112] Liu QL, Zhang J, Liu X, Gao JY. Role of growth hormone in maturation and activation of dendritic cells via miR-200a and the Keap1/Nrf2 pathway. Cell Proliferation. 2015;**48**:573-581. DOI: 10.1111/cpr.12206

[113] Weigent DA, Blalock JE, LeBoeuf RD. An antisense oligodeoxynucleotide to growth hormone messenger ribonucleic acid inhibits lymphocyte proliferation. Endocrinology. 1991;**128**:2053-2057. DOI: 10.1210/endo-128-4-2053

[114] Baxter JB, Blalock JE, Weigent DA. Characterization of immunoreactive insulin-like growth factor-I from leukocytes and its regulation by growth hormone. Endocrinology. 1991;**129**:1727-1734. DOI: 10.1210/endo-129-4-1727

[115] Arnold RE, Weigent DA. The inhibition of superoxide production in EL4 lymphoma cells overexpressing growth hormone. Immunopharmacology and Immunotoxicology. 2003;**25**:159-177. DOI: 10.1081/IPH-120020467

[116] Arnold RE, Weigent DA. The production of nitric oxide in EL4 lymphoma cells overexpressing growth hormone. Journal of Neuroimmunology. 2003;**134**:82-94. DOI: 10.1016/S0165-5728(02)00420-4

[117] Arnold RE, Weigent DA. The inhibition of apoptosis in EL4 lymphoma cells overexpressing growth hormone. Neuroimmunomodulation. 2004;**11**:149-159. DOI: 10.1159/000076764

[118] Weigent DA, Arnold RE. Expression of insulin-like growth factor-1 and insulin-like growth factor-1 receptors in EL4 lymphoma cells overexpressing growth hormone. Cellular Immunology. 2005;**234**:54-66. DOI: 10.1016/j.cellimm.2005.04.016

[119] Farmer JT, Weigent DA. Expression of insulin-like growth factor-2 receptors on EL4 cells overexpressing growth hormone. Brain, Behavior, and Immunity. 2007;**21**:79-85. DOI: 10.1016/j.bbi.2006.02.006

[120] Farmer JT, Weigent DA. TGF-beta1 expression in EL4 lymphoma cells overexpressing growth hormone. Cellular Immunology. 2006;**240**:22-30. DOI: 10.1016/j.cellimm.2006.06.003

[121] Weigent DA. Regulation of Id2 expression in EL4 T lymphoma cells overexpressing growth hormone. Cellular Immunology. 2009;**255**:46-54. DOI: 10.1016/j.cellimm.2008.10.003

[122] Malarkey WB, Wang J, Cheney C, Glaser R, Nagaraja H. Human lymphocyte growth hormone stimulates interferon gamma production and is inhibited by cortisol and norepinephrine. Journal of Neuroimmunology. 2002;**123**:180-187. DOI: 10.1016/S0165-5728(01)00489-1

[123] Re RN, Cook JL. Senescence, apoptosis, and stem cell biology: The rationale for an expanded view of intracrine action. American Journal of Physiology. Heart and Circulatory Physiology. 2009;**297**:H893-H901. DOI: 10.1152/ajpheart.00414.2009

[124] Weigent DA. High molecular weight isoforms of growth hormone In cells of the immune system. Cellular Immunology. 2011;**271**:44-52. DOI: 10.1016/j.cellimm.2011.06.001

[125] Caballero-Villarraso J, Aguado R, Cañete MD, Roldán L, Cañete R, Santamaría M. Hormone replacement therapy in children with growth hormone deficiency: Iimpact on immune profile. Archives of Physiology and Biochemistry. 2019;**19**:1-5. DOI: 10.1080//13813455.2019.1628070

[126] Lebi J, Sediva A, Snajderova M, Pruhova S, Rakoskinova V. Immune system in adults with childhood-onset growth hormone deficiency: Effect of growth hormone therapy. Endocrine Regulations. 2000;**34**:169-173

[127] Rekers-Mombarg LT, Rijkers GT, Massa GG, Wit JM. Immunologic studies in children with idiopathic short-stature before and during growth hormone therapy. Dutch growth hormone working group. Hormone Research. 1995;**44**:203-207. DOI: 10.1159/000184626

[128] Spadoni GL, Rossi P, Ragno W, Galli E, Cianfarani S, Galasso C, et al. Immune function in growth hormone-deficient children treated with biosynthetic growth hormone. Acta Paediatrica Scandinavica. 1991;**80**:75-79. DOI: 10.1111/j.1651-2227.1991.tb11733.x

[129] Höybye C, Faseh L, Himonakos C, Pielak T, Eugen-Olsen P. Serum soluble urokinase plasminogen activator receptor (suPAR) in adults with growth hormone deficiency. Endocrine Connections. 2019;**8**:772-779. DOI: 10.1530/EC-19-0159

[130] Lobie PE, Breipohl W, Waters MJ. Growth hormone receptor expression in the rat gastrointestinal tract. Endocrinology. 1990;**126**:299-306. DOI: 10.1210/endo-126-1-299

[131] Lincoln DT, Kaiser HE, Raju GP, Waters MJ. Growth hormone expression and colorectal carcinoma: Localization of receptors. In Vivo. 2000;**14**:41-49

[132] Gilbert S, Zhang R, Denson L, Moriggi R, Steinbrecher K, Shroyer N, et al. Enterocyte STAT5 promotes mucosal wound healing via suppression of myosin light chain kinase-mediated loss of barrier function and inflammation. EMBO Molecular Medicine. 2012;**4**:109-124. DOI: 10.1002/emmm.201100192

[133] Han X, Ren X, Jurickova I, Groschwitz K, Pasternak BA, Xu H, et al. Regulation of intestinal barrier function by signal transducer and activator of transcription 5b. Gut. 2009;**58**:49-58. DOI: 10.1136/gut.2007.145094

[134] Soendergaard C, Kvist PH, Thygesen P, Reslow M, Nielsen OH, Kopchil JJ, et al. Characterization of growth hormone resistance in experimental and ulcerative colitis. International Journal of Molecular Sciences. 2017;**18**:2046. DOI: 10.3390/ijms18102046

[135] Devesa J, Devesa P, Reimunde P. Growth hormone revisited. Medicina Clínica (Barcelona). 2010;**135**:665-670. DOI: 10.1016/j.medcli.2009.10.017

[136] Balducci R, Toscano V, Larizza D, Mangiantini A, Gaiasso C, Municchi G, et al. Effects of long-term growth hormone therapy on adrenal steroidogenesis in turner syndrome. Hormone Research. 1998;**49**:210-215. DOI: 10.1159/000023173

[137] Isidori AM, Kaltsas GA, Perry L, Burrin JM, Besser GM, Monson JP. The effect of growth hormone replacement therapy on adrenal androgen secretion in adult onset hypopituitarism. Clinical Endocrinology. 2003;**58**:601-611. DOI: 10.1046/j.1365-2265.2003.01759.x

[138] Ciresi A, Radellini S, Vigneri E, Guarnotta V, Bianco J, Mineo MG, et al. Correlation between adrenal function, growth hormone secretion, and insulin sensitivity in children with idiopathic growth hormone deficiency. Journal of Endocrinological Investigation. 2018;**41**:333-342. DOI: 10.1007/s40618-017-0747-2

[139] Devaskar UP, Devaskar SU, Voina S, Velayo N, Sperling MA. Growth hormone stimulates adrenal steroidogenesis in the fetus. Nature. 1981;**290**:404-405. DOI: 10.1038/290404a0

[140] McFarlane AC, Edmondson SR, Wintour EM, Werther GA. GH-receptor distribution in the ovine foetal adrenal gland: Ontogenic and functional studies. The Journal of Endocrinology. 1999;**162**:197-205. DOI: 10.1677/joe.0.1620197

[141] Li Y, Zhang Y, Zhang M, Yang W, Ji B, Pan H, et al. Growth hormone peak modifies the effect of BMI on increased systolic blood pressure in children with short stature. Scientific Reports. 2019;**9**:7879. DOI: 10.1038/s41598-019-44299-9

[142] Butler G, Turlejski T, Wales G, Bailey L, Wright N. Growth hormone treatment and health-related quality of life in children and adolescents: A national, prospective, one-year controlled study. Clinical Endocrinology. 2019;**91**:304-313. DOI: 10.1111/cen.14011

[143] Butler T, Harvey P, Cardozo L, Zhu YS, Mosa A, Tanzi E, et al. Epilepsy, depression, and growth hormone. Epilepsy & Behavior. 2019;**94**:297-300. DOI: 10.1016/j.yebeh.2019.01.022

[144] Ford ZK, Dourson AJ, Liu X, Lu P, Green KJ, Hudgins RC, et al. Systemic growth hormone deficiency causes mechanical and thermal hypersensitivity during early postnatal development. IBRO Report. 2019;**6**:111-121. DOI: 10.1016/j.ibror.2019.02.001

[145] Hu Y, Liu X, Chen X, Chen T, Ye P, Jiang L, et al. Differences in the functional connectivity density of the brain between individuals with growth hormone deficiency and idiopathic short stature. Psychoneuroendocrinology. 2019;**103**:67-75. DOI: 10.1016/j.psyneuen.2018.12.229

Chapter 4

Fetal Growth Restriction

Edurne Mazarico Gallego, Ariadna Torrecillas Pujol,
Alex Joan Cahuana Bartra and
Maria Dolores Gómez Roig

Additional information is available at the end of the chapter

http://dx.doi.org/10.5772/intechopen.90712

Abstract

Fetal growth defect is classified into intrauterine growth restriction (IUGR) and small-for-gestational-age (SGA) fetus based on the estimated fetal weight percentile and Doppler hemodynamic parameters. IUGR pathophysiology and etiology are complex and diverse, highlighting placental insufficiency as a paradigm, which explains its association with other entities of great clinical importance such as preeclampsia. The poor long- and short-term perinatal and postnatal results associated with this context make it necessary to establish an early diagnosis and a therapeutic strategy, which can be challenging due to the compromise between the threat of intrauterine permanence and the prematurity problem. Consequently, a systematic and protocolized diagnostic-therapeutic management, based on scientific evidence, is necessary to determine whether obstetric intervention through a preterm delivery is advisable to improve the perinatal outcomes of these patients.

Keywords: fetal growth, intrauterine growth restriction, small-for-gestational-age fetus, Doppler evaluation, prematurity

1. Introduction

In general terms, fetal growth defect is considered the impossibility of achieving the genetically determined potential size [1]. In the vast majority of cases, it is related to uteroplacental insufficiency in the context of intrauterine growth restriction (IUGR). Despite its origin remains unknown, it is believed to be caused by an interaction of environmental and genetic factors with either a fetal, placental, or maternal origin. Various complications are associated with IUGR; these may include stillbirth, prematurity, neonatal morbi-mortality, endocrine and metabolic alterations, increased cardiovascular risk, and long-term neurological sequelae [2].

IntechOpen

© 2020 The Author(s). Licensee IntechOpen. This chapter is distributed under the terms of the Creative Commons Attribution License (http://creativecommons.org/licenses/by/3.0), which permits unrestricted use, distribution, and reproduction in any medium, provided the original work is properly cited. (cc) BY

IUGR fetus identification is one of the main objectives of prenatal care, since proper perinatal diagnosis and management reduces perinatal morbi-mortality [3]. Most small fetuses are not diagnosed during pregnancy [4], not even in high-risk subpopulations. This is in part due to the large number of reference tables used and the lack of international standards comparable to those for child growth [5]. Therefore, it is necessary to improve the prenatal diagnosis of these cases. With this purpose, it is essential to have an agreed definition between obstetricians and neonatologists, which would allow to compare data, to conduct prospective studies, and to analyze results between different institutions [2].

2. Definitions

Fetal growth defect (FGD) is defined as an ultrasound estimated fetal weight (EFW) below the 10th percentile for gestational age and gender [2].

Among FGD fetuses, Doppler hemodynamic evaluation differentiates fetuses with higher risk of perinatal morbi-mortality [6]. Hence, fetal growth restriction definition incorporates the Doppler hemodynamic evaluation to distinguish the fetuses with placental involvement from those without that affectation. These unaffected fetuses have a better prognosis and are known as small-for-gestational-age (SGA) fetuses [2].

Fetal weight estimation is based on Hadlock's formula which includes biparietal diameter (BPD), head circumference (HC), abdominal circumference (AC), and femur length (FL) [7]. However, there is controversy about fetal weight percentile estimation in the medical literature. Percentile customization according to maternal and/or paternal features is one of the main sources of heterogeneity in the IUGR definition. The utility of customized percentiles is to a certain extent limited because factors used for customization are not powerful predictors of birth weight [8]. Maternal height, weight, and ethnicity/race are related to fetal size but do not explain the important variability in birth weight. Thus, the limitations of these parameters restrict their usefulness for IUGR definition [2]. For that reason, the Fetal Growth Longitudinal Study, part of the Intergrowth-21st Project, aimed to develop international tabulated standards for fetal growth [9]. These curves have the advantage of using fetal growth standards derived from healthy populations. This reduces the underdiagnosis that may occur when fetal growth is contrasted against references including the high-risk mothers. At the various study sites, these curves have proven to be similar for all fetal and newborn measurements showing the same growth potential regardless of the race [10]. Thus, the reported differences were probably related to nutritional problems rather than geographical location or ethnicity [2]. However, several subsequent studies have shown that individualized fetal growth tables improve the identification of patients at risk of adverse perinatal outcomes [11].

2.1. Differences between IUGR and SGA

A small fetus is associated with worse obstetric results. At least two groups of small fetuses are distinguished: IUGR and SGA [2]. **Table 1** shows its main differences:

http://dx.doi.org/10.5772/intechopen.90712

	IUGR	SGA
Perinatal outcomes	Worse	Similar to normal fetuses
Growth delay	"True"	"Constitutional"
Doppler ultrasound	Hemodynamic redistribution	Normal
Abnormal environment adaptation	Present	Absent
Preeclampsia risk	Higher	Lower

Table 1. Differences between IUGR and SGA.

IUGR term refers to small fetuses with a higher risk of intrauterine fetal deterioration, stillbirth, and, in general, a worse perinatal outcome than those with normal growth. These fetuses have a "true" growth delay and are generally associated with Doppler ultrasound signs which suggest hemodynamic redistribution due to an adaptation to fetal malnutrition/hypoxia with histological and biochemical signs of placental disease. IUGR is also associated with an increased risk of preeclampsia [2].

2.2. IUGR vs. SGA definition

Current evidence suggests that there is no superior parameter for differentiating IUGR from SGA [2]. As for the individual Doppler ultrasound study, the best candidate is the cerebroplacental ratio (CPR), which is calculated dividing the middle cerebral artery (MCA) Doppler pulsatility index (PI) (MCA-PI) by the umbilical artery (UA) Doppler PI (UA-PI). This ratio reflects small decreases in fetal cerebral vascular resistance with slight increases in placental resistance in a combined way. This relationship seems to be more sensitive to hypoxia than its individual components, correlating better with a possible adverse outcome [12]. The uterine artery (UtA) PI (UtA-PI) is a predictor of worse perinatal results in small fetuses [13]. Another poor outcome predictive factor is a very small EFW regardless of the CPR and the UtA-PI values. An EFW below the 3rd percentile indicates a much higher risk of adverse perinatal outcomes [14]. Therefore, when there are any of the three parameters mentioned above (CPR, UtA-PI, and/or EFW < 3rd percentile), the risk of adverse perinatal outcomes increases. For this reason, the definition of IUGR must include these three parameters [2].

Summarizing the definition [2, 15]:

- A SGA fetus is defined as an EFW lower than the 10th percentile and greater than or equal to the 3rd percentile for gestational age and gender with a normal Doppler hemodynamic study.
- An IUGR is defined as:
    - An EFW below the 3rd percentile for gestational age and gender
    - An EFW below the 10th percentile for gestational age and gender plus an altered Doppler hemodynamic study

2.3. Severe early onset vs. moderate late onset IUGR

The IUGR is presented in two different phenotypes according to disease onset time during pregnancy: early onset IUGR and late onset IUGR. Generally, there is a correlation between early onset and more severe IUGR forms, so two types of IUGR are defined: severe early onset and moderate late onset. The cutoff point for these forms has been arbitrarily established at 32 weeks [2]. In **Table 2**, we observe the differences between both clinical forms.

2.3.1. Severe early onset IUGR

The severe early onset IUGR represents 20–30% of all IUGR. It is related to severe placental insufficiency and chronic fetal hypoxia, and so UA Doppler is often pathological [16]. In this context, this type of IUGR is associated with early preeclampsia in up to 50% of cases [17] and with severe damage and/or stillbirth before term [18]. Besides, its clinical management is a challenge due to the necessity to balance the risks of intrauterine permanence with the complications derived from prematurity [2].

Without treatment, fetal well-being deteriorates with a progression toward hypoxia and acidosis, which is reflected in the sequence of alterations of the UA Doppler and the PI of the ductus venosus (DV). The latency period to severe fetal deterioration is variable, but it usually lasts for weeks [19] and depends on the severity of the placental compromise. The sequence of changes (**Figure 1**) is relatively constant, especially in the signs of advanced stages, except in the cases where there is an associated preeclampsia which can distort the natural history. In such cases, fetal deterioration might appear unexpectedly. These changes in fetal Doppler allow for the monitorization of the progression of fetal deterioration and the scheduling of the delivery in an elective manner [2].

		Severe early-onset IUGR	**Moderate late-onset IUGR**
IUGR %		20-30%	70-80%
Prevalence		1-2% (low)	3-5% (high)
Problem		Management	Diagnosis
Placental disease	**Intensity**	Severe	Moderate
	UA Doppler	Altered	Normal
	Preeclampsia association	High	Low
Hypoxia		++	+/-
Cardiovascular adaptation		Systemic	Central
Fetal Maturity		Immature fetus	Mature fetus
Hypoxia tolerance		High	Low
Natural history of fetal deterioration		Present	Absent (or fast evolution)
Morbi-mortality		High	Low (but common stillbirth cause). Adverse long-term outcomes

Table 2. Differences between severe early-onset IUGR vs. moderate late-onset IUGR (adapted from Ref. [2]).

http://dx.doi.org/10.5772/intechopen.90712

2.3.2. Moderate late onset IUGR

These fetuses represent 70–80% of cases [17]. The placental alteration is mild, and, therefore, the UA is generally normal [20] and there is low association with preeclampsia (10%) [17]. In these cases, the diagnostic rates are low, and that is what makes the late (undiagnosed) IUGR to contribute in a large proportion of late stillbirth [21].

In moderate lateonset IUGR, there is a high rate of CPR alteration [20]. In addition, in 25% of cases of late onset IUGR, a cerebral vasodilation may occur (MCA-PI below the 5th percentile), reflecting a situation of chronic hypoxia. Besides, signs of advanced fetal deterioration with changes in the ductus venosus are hardly ever observed [20]. For this reason, the sequential fetal deterioration cascade described previously does not occur (**Figure 2**). These fetuses may suffer rapid deterioration which can lead to serious injury or death. The explanation behind this fact could be a combination of factors such as the low tolerance of preterm fetuses to hypoxia (compared to preterm fetuses), the higher frequency of uterine contractions in term gestations, and some cases of acute placental failure [2]. Despite the benign nature of this type of fetus, the risk of acute fetal deterioration before delivery significantly contributes to late stillbirth [22] and to a high association with intrapartum fetal distress and neonatal acidosis [23].

2.3.3. Common problems

Both IUGR types are associated with a worse long-term prognosis in neurological, cardiovascular, and metabolic development [24–27]. This would mean that, regardless of severity, chronic exposure to an adverse intrauterine environment is essential to develop adverse fetal programming. Predictably, different stages of fetal maturation would determine different adaptive programming responses [2].

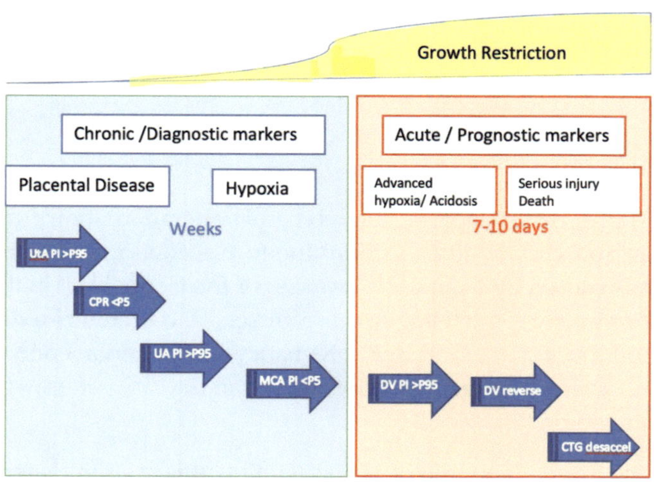

Figure 1. Sequence of changes in severe early-onset IUGR. Adapted from Ref. [2].

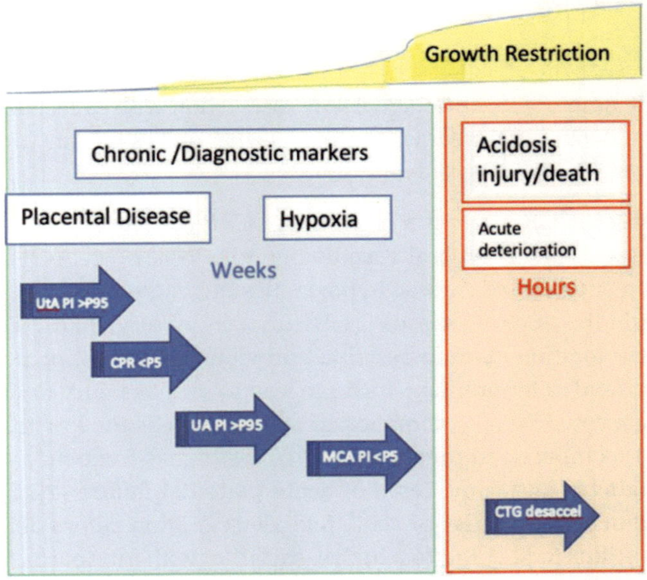

Figure 2. Sequence of changes of moderate late-onset IUGR. Adapted from Ref. [2].

The evidence suggests that both early and late onset IUGR are a consequence of a placental disease, but it is unknown to what extent they are the same type of pathology. Placental insufficiency of early onset IUGR is associated with histological signs of alteration in early implantation [28]. It is not clear, however, if late IUGR is a mild form of abnormal placental implantation at the beginning of the pregnancy or if it is an added placental damage produced in the second half of pregnancy. The latter option would be supported by the fact that part of these patients has abnormal UtA Doppler in the third trimester being this one previously normal [29].

3. Etiology

3.1. Placental disease

In general terms, IUGR with Doppler hemodynamic alteration shows fetal adaptation to a hypoxia situation and chronic malnutrition due to placental insufficiency. This placental function alteration is caused by a deficient invasion of the trophoblast in the maternal spiral arteries, with an incomplete remodeling of these vessels, and therefore a deficit in the physiological vasodilation that occurs in normal pregnancy. This phenomenon can be monitored by assessing uterine artery resistance, which increases in the cases of growth restriction associated with placental origin [2].

It is likely that in the future, biomarkers of placental insufficiency in maternal blood may be incorporated as a diagnostic criterion for IUGR as markers of placental involvement in this pathology. Recent evidence suggests that angiogenic factors predict a poor perinatal outcome in small fetuses, with predictive values similar to CPR and UtA Doppler, but without a proven additive value [30]. An increase in anti-angiogenic factors sFlt1 and soluble endoglin (sEnd) and a decrease in pro-angiogenic factors (placental growth factor—PGF) have been observed.

3.2. Infectious disease

Cytomegalovirus: it is the first cause of congenital infection in Europe (0.3–0.6%). Most cases are asymptomatic. The risk of congenital disease is higher if the infection occurs during the first and second trimesters. In contrast, the transmission risk increases in the third trimester, but fetuses infected at this time are generally born healthy [31].

Congenital varicella: it is more frequent when the maternal disease is acquired between 8 and 20 weeks of gestation. Very rare fetal involvement is observed in the second and third trimesters. There is an affectation of the musculoskeletal system and an affectation of the autonomic nervous system [32].

Congenital rubella: there is a higher incidence of the disease in developing countries [33]. Fetal involvement is observed in the vast majority of cases in which maternal infection occurs in the first trimester, being infrequent beyond 17 weeks.

HIV: a relationship between HIV seropositivity and the increased risk of spontaneous abortion, stillbirth, IUGR, low birth weight, premature delivery, and neurodevelopmental alteration [34] has been observed. The association between premature birth and low birth weight has also been related to the use of highly active antiretroviral therapy (HAART) [35]. In these patients, an increased risk of placental insufficiency has been described [36].

Malaria: this infection causes a massive sequestration of erythrocytes in the syncytiotrophoblast. Multiple mechanisms contribute to fetal growth restriction, including abnormal vascularization, impaired growth hormone expression, difficulty in transporting nutrients, and a process of inflammation and activation of the immune response [37].

3.3. Genetic disorders

Only 2% of the cases with fetal growth restriction without structural abnormalities are associated with alterations in the karyotype [38]. The risk of a genetic syndrome with cognitive repercussion is increased if there are malformations, microcephaly, and/or progressive flattening of biometrics.

3.4. External factors

Smoking is the main contributor to fetal growth restriction in our environment. The odds ratio for developing IUGR in pregnant smokers is 1.9 (95% confidence interval (CI): 1.69–2.13). The risk is directly proportional to consumption [39].

4. Fetal well-being assessment

Fetal well-being assessment is based on determining whether the fetus is suffering from any chronic affectation (due to a progressive increase in hypoxemia and/or hypoxia) or an acute involvement (acute changes in advanced stages of fetal compromise, characterized by severe hypoxia and metabolic acidosis) whose alteration usually precedes fetal death within a few days.

UA Doppler: it is the only measure that provides both diagnostic and prognostic information for IUGR management. The progression of the Doppler patterns of the UA toward an absent or reverse diastolic flow correlates with the risk of fetal injury or death [2].

MCA Doppler: it reports the presence of cerebral vasodilation, a subrogated hypoxia biomarker. Its alteration is considered a late manifestation. Fetuses with an altered MCA-PI have a six times higher risk of urgent cesarean section due to suspected loss of fetal well-being than fetuses with a normal PI [40].

CPR: it has mainly a diagnostic value. It significantly improves the sensitivity of the UA and the isolated MCA, since the increase in placental impedance (UA-PI) is usually combined with a decrease in brain resistance (MCA-PI) [41].

Ductus venosus (DV) Doppler: it is the parameter that, by itself, has the greatest capacity to predict the risk of short-term stillbirth in early onset IUGR. The absent/reverse flow during atrial contraction is associated with perinatal mortality, regardless of gestational age [42], with a risk ranging from 40 to 100% in the cases of early onset IUGR [43].

Aortic isthmus (AoI) Doppler: it is associated with an increase in fetal mortality and neurological morbidity in the cases of early onset IUGR. This vessel reflects the balance between cerebral impedance and the systemic vascular system [44]. Longitudinal studies show that alterations in AoI precede those of DV in 1 week [45] and, therefore, it is not a good predictor of short-term stillbirth risk. In contrast, AoI seems to improve the prediction of neurological morbidity [46].

Uterine artery Doppler (UtA): the study of the uterine artery flow has mainly focused on predicting the risk of preeclampsia and fetal growth restriction. However, this flow has also been considered both as diagnostic and fetal well-being assessment tool in SGA fetuses. There is a statistically significant correlation among the Doppler alteration in the UA, the Doppler alteration in the UtA, and an adverse perinatal outcome. Both vessels are comparable in their prediction ability [43].

Computerized cardiotocography (CTG): it provided with new knowledge about the pathophysiology and management of IUGR. It evaluates the short-term variability (STV) of fetal heart rate, a parameter that cannot be subjectively evaluated. Current evidence suggests that computerized CTG is sensitive for the detection of advanced fetal impairment, and that provides a value similar to that of DV with a reverse atrial flow for the prediction of short-term fetal death. A low variability of fetal heart rate is correlated with the presence of acidosis and severe hypoxia, a fact that has been demonstrated with cord blood collected at the time of cesarean section. Despite the high implementation of conventional CTG in all clinical control protocols, it has not been shown to reduce mortality in high-risk pregnancies given its high inter- and intra-observer variability in interpretation [47].

Biophysical profile (BPP): it is obtained by combining ultrasound evaluation of fetal tone, respiratory movements, and body movements with amniotic fluid and conventional CTG. A systematic review [48] found that the use of BPP does not reduce perinatal mortality (relative risk (RR) 1.33, 95% CI 0.60–2.98) or APGAR less than 7 at 5 min (RR 1.27, 95% CI 0.85–1.92). An increased risk of cesarean section was also found (RR 1.60, 95% CI 1.05–2.44). It is currently not recommended to perform a BPP for the control of the preterm SGA fetus.

Amniotic fluid index (AFI): it is basically used as part of the BPP. There is limited evidence on the role of oligoamnios as a predictor of perinatal complications in IUGR fetuses with Doppler follow-up, its inclusion being questionable in management protocols [2].

5. Diagnosis

5.1. Clinical diagnosis

Uterine height will be performed at each visit from 26 weeks. The methodology will be supine position, from fundus to pubis, and masked observation of the previous exploration. If the uterine height is less than the 10th percentile for gestational age and no EFW is available in the previous 2 weeks, an ultrasound EFW is required.

5.2. Ultrasound diagnosis

Fetal weight estimation requires three steps:

- First step: gestation dating according to crown-rump length.
- Second step: calculation of EFW according to fetal biometrics—algorithm that includes BPD, HC, AC, and FL [49]. If the cephalic measurements are not valuable, an alternative algorithm with FL and AC will be used [50].
- Third step: calculation of the growth percentile according to reference tables.

5.3. Diagnosis of the type of alteration

5.3.1. Study protocol

Detailed anamnesis:

- Toxic habits: tobacco, alcohol, drugs, medication, and work [51]
- Maternal and paternal weight and size, weight of the patient at birth, and measurement of blood pressure (BP) at the beginning of pregnancy
- Sexual history of the couple: relationship time. Type of contraception. Artificial fertilization techniques
- Previous obstetric clinical history: neonatal weight of previous children (the history of a previous SGA doubles the risk in successive pregnancies) [52], history of fetal death, preeclampsia, growth restriction, repeated abortions, placental abruption, and premature deliveries [15]

- Medical history: diabetes with vascular disease, moderate and severe nephropathy, cyanotic congenital heart disease, arterial hypertension, antiphospholipid syndrome, and systemic lupus erythematosus [53]

Maternal physical examination: weight, height, uterine height, limb examination in search of chronic vascular disease, blood pressure.

Complementary explorations:

- **Ultrasound:** detailed anatomical assessment. 20–60% of congenital malformations are accompanied by growth disturbance [54], and approximately 10% of fetuses with growth restriction have an associated congenital anomaly [55]. It is also important to assess Doppler study (UA, MCA, UtA, and CPR), placenta, amniotic fluid, and chromosomopathy markers.
- **Neurosonography and echocardiography**: for a growth below the 3rd percentile.
- Proteinuria study.
- **Complete blood test** with hemogram, coagulation, and basal biochemistry (with liver and kidney profile).
- **Amniocentesis:** it is advisable to perform an amniocentesis to rule out chromosomal abnormalities when the diagnosis of IUGR is made at early gestational ages. The rate of chromosomal abnormalities in IUGR fetuses is approximately 20% if diagnosed before 23 weeks, being practically null afterward [56]. Genetic studies in amniotic fluid are recommendable if any of the following criteria is met:
    - Quantitative fluorescence-polymerase chain reaction (QF-PCR) and molecular karyotype (array CGH):
    - IUGR diagnosis prior to 24 weeks and severe (below the 3rd percentile)
    - IUGR diagnosis prior to 28 weeks and severe (below the 3rd percentile) accompanied by ultrasound markers (excluding oligoamnios), minor structural anomaly, or biometrics (FL or HC) < −3 standard deviations (SD)
    - EFW lower than the 10th percentile accompanied by any major structural anomaly
    - Study of bone alterations (add it to QF-PCR and molecular karyotype)
    - Achondroplasia and hypochondroplasia study if bone biometrics < −3 SD or femur/foot ratio < 0.85.
    - Genetic counseling to assess skeletal dysplasia study if malformations associated with dysplasia, bone morphological alterations (fractures, curvatures, hypomineralization), or long bone length below the 1st percentile.
    - Study of specific genetic panels or exome sequencing (request genetic counseling to assess these studies)

http://dx.doi.org/10.5772/intechopen.90712

- If IUGR with more than one structural anomaly of two systems (except hypospadias) of high syndromic risk
- Biometrics (FL or HC) < −4 SD with no signs of placental insufficiency and normal molecular karyotype result

- **Infections study:** it is estimated that around 5% of SGA fetuses have an infectious cause. The most frequently implicated pathogen is CMV, followed by toxoplasma and syphilis [2]. Facing IUGR diagnosis, it is necessary to request:
  - Rubella study.
  - Syphilis study: treponemal and reaginic test in maternal blood.
  - Malaria study: for populations at risk (from endemic areas) [57].
  - CMV study: in the case of indication of invasive technique, it is necessary to perform CMV PCR in amniotic fluid. In the case of non-indication of invasive technique, maternal serologies (IgG and IgM) will be requested only in IUGR (excludes SGA). If IgG and IgM are negative, the infection is discarded. If IgG and IgM are positive, it is recommended to perform an amniocentesis for CMV PCR in amniotic fluid. If IgG is positive but IgM is negative, it is advisable to perform an amniocentesis only if there is an ultrasound marker compatible with CMV infection (except an isolated oligoamnios).

5.3.2. Classification

IUGR is classified into stages, as shown in **Table 3**:

Stage	Pathophysiological Correlation	Criteria
I	Very small EFW or moderate placental insufficiency	EFW < p3 EFW < p10 + any of these criteria: • CPR < p5* • PI MCA < p5* • PI UtA > p95
II	Severe placental insufficiency	EFW < p10 + absent diastolic flow in UA**
III	Low suspicion of fetal acidosis	EFW < p10 + any of these criteria: • Reverse diastolic flow in UA** • PI-DV > p95 or absent diastolic flow in the DV***
IV	High suspicion of fetal acidosis	EFW < p10 + any of these criteria: • Reverse diastolic flow in the DV*** • Pathological CTG

*on two separated occasions > 12h.
** > 50% of cycles, in free cord loop in both arteries on two separated occasions > 12h.
*** on two separated occasions > 6-12h.

Table 3. IUGR stages (adapted from Refs. [2, 15]).

5.4. Follow-up

Follow-up visits for Doppler study will be adapted to the degree of fetal involvement [15]:

- SGA: control every 2–3 weeks
- IUGR stage I: control every 1–2 weeks
- IUGR stage II: control every 2–4 days
- IUGR stage III: control every 24–48 h
- IUGR stage IV: control every 12–48 h

During visits, Doppler control and CTG will be carried out. EFW assessment will be carried out at intervals equal to or greater than 15 days. When IUGR is accompanied by severe preeclampsia, the follow-up should correspond to the follow-up of the immediately superior IUGR stage.

6. Obstetric behavior

6.1. Prenatal obstetric behavior

6.1.1. General recommendations

- Avoid complete rest, as it does not improve fetal growth or perinatal outcome [58].
- Promote the elimination of possible external factors, such as tobacco. Quitting smoking reduces the risk of having SGA fetus. Although the benefit is greater if tobacco is abandoned before 15 weeks [59], smoking cessation should be advised when diagnosing SGA fetus at any gestational age [60].
- Work leave is advisable [15].
- Lung maturation only if termination criteria are met and gestational age is greater than 26 weeks (26–34.6 weeks).
- The criteria for neuroprophylaxis with magnesium sulfate will be <34 weeks and whenever possible >4 h before birth.

6.1.2 Termination of pregnancy: gestational age and delivery

The optimal moment of termination requires a balance between the risks of prematurity with those of intrauterine permanence (death and multiple organ damage due to inadequate tissue perfusion) [61]. The objective of IUGR vigilance is to evaluate fetal and neonatal risks to optimize intervention times, as well as to choose the best route of delivery. **Table 4** shows the recommended gestational age and delivery according to fetal growth defect.

http://dx.doi.org/10.5772/intechopen.90712

	Gestational age	Delivery
SGA	≥ 40 gestation weeks	Vaginal delivery not contraindicated
IUGR stage I	≥ 37 gestation weeks	Vaginal delivery not contraindicated (If MCA-PI < p5, the risk of urgent caesarean section is 50%)
IUGR stage II	≥ 34 gestation weeks	Elective caesarean section
IUGR stage III	≥ 30 gestation weeks	
IUGR stage IV	≥ 26 gestation weeks	

Table 4. Recommended gestational age and delivery according to fetal growth defect.

Depending on the gestational age when we proceed to termination, we will have various degrees of prematurity:

- Extreme prematurity (24–28 weeks). In this period, each additional day of pregnancy represents an increase of 1–2% in the chances of survival [2]. Less than 26 weeks will be considered in the periviable infant with chances of survival without severe sequelae below 50% [15].
- Moderate prematurity (28–34 weeks). The presence of reverse flow in the umbilical artery is associated with a RR of 10.6 for the development of perinatal morbi-mortality [2].
- Late prematurity (34–36 weeks). There is not neither a high mortality rate nor severe morbidity, but there is a worse perinatal and cognitive outcome [62]. The decrease in diastolic velocities of the umbilical artery correlates with fetal nutritional deterioration [63] and its neurodevelopment [64]. The fetus with absent telediastolic flow of the umbilical artery presents four times greater risk of severe morbidity and perinatal mortality [65].
- Full-term gestation (>37 weeks). Cerebral hemodynamic redistribution is associated with worse perinatal and cognitive outcome [13].

Labor in fetuses with growth restriction is associated with an increase in the rate of urgent cesarean sections. Therefore, in the presence of signs of severe fetal deterioration such as absent or reverse umbilical diastolic flow, an elective cesarean section is advised.

6.1.3. Termination methods

Cervical maturation will begin with a PGE2 slow-release device, mechanical methods, or oxytocic induction depending on cervical conditions and uterine dynamics [66].

6.2. Intrapartum obstetric behavior

Continuous monitoring is necessary and an adequate resuscitation according to the baby's weight. It is also important to carry out a placental anatomo-pathological study in all cases.

6.3. Postpartum obstetric behavior

6.3.1. Immediate postpartum

- Protein/creatinine ratio and hepatic and renal profile: in those cases not studied prenatally and with IUGR criteria [15].
- CMV maternal serologies (IgG): to perform breast milk processing before administration and to avoid vertical transmission. It should be carried out in those cases with no prenatal studies and with IUGR criteria with delivery before 32 weeks or birth weight below 1500 g.

6.3.2. Quarantine

- Thrombophilic study: early onset IUGR, preeclampsia, or placental abruption.
- Explanation of the anatomo-pathological report of placenta. The massive deposit of perivillositary fibrin is associated with a risk of recurrence of 40–60%. The patient should be informed of the possibility of prophylaxis with heparin in a subsequent pregnancy to reduce this risk.

7. Conclusion

FGD is an important cause of perinatal morbidity. Its diagnosis, management, and monitoring according to clinical evidence are very important to improve perinatal outcomes in these cases.

7.1. Recommendation and future directions

1. It is very important to improve the diagnosis of fetuses with FGD. For this reason, the first trimester ultrasound is essential to date the pregnancy correctly. A second trimester ultrasound should be performed to detect fetal anomalies and to detect the most severe and early cases of FGD and a third trimester ultrasound to increase the diagnosis of late FGD.
2. In those cases with risk factors for growth defects, additional ultrasounds are recommended in the third trimester.
3. A careful etiological diagnosis should be done to rule out malformations, infections, or genetic alterations.
4. The management and follow-up of these gestations must be based on systematic protocols based on clinical evidence that facilitate the unification of clinical practice.

Abbreviations

IUGR	intrauterine growth restriction
SGA	small for gestational age

http://dx.doi.org/10.5772/intechopen.90712

FGD	fetal growth defect
EFW	estimated fetal weight
BPD	biparietal diameter
HC	head circumference
AC	abdominal circumference
FL	femur length
CPR	cerebroplacental ratio
MCA	middle cerebral artery
PI	pulsatility index
UA	umbilical artery
UtA	uterine artery
HIV	human immunodeficiency virus
HAART	highly active antiretroviral therapy
DV	ductus venosus
CTG	computerized cardiotocography
BPP	biophysical profile
STV	short-term variability
RR	relative risk
CI	confidence interval
AFI	amniotic fluid index
BP	blood pressure
QF-PCR	quantitative fluorescence-polymerase chain reaction
PCR	polymerase chain reaction
SD	standard deviation
IgG	immunoglobulin G
IgM	immunoglobulin M
PGE_2	prostaglandin E_2

Author details

Edurne Mazarico Gallego*, Ariadna Torrecillas Pujol, Alex Joan Cahuana Bartra and Maria Dolores Gómez Roig

*Address all correspondence to: emazarico@sjdhospitalbarcelona.org

Hospital Sant Joan de Deu and Hospital Clínic, BCNatal-Barcelona Center for Maternal-Fetal and Neonatal Medicine, Barcelona, Spain

References

[1] Gomez MD, Garcia-Algar O. Crecimiento intrauterino restringido: ¿problema de definicion o de contenido? Anales de Pediatría (Barcelona, Spain). 2011;**75**:157-160

[2] Gomez MD, Llurba E, Gratacos E, Oros D, Garcia O, Rodriguez G. Defectos del crecimiento fetal. Documento de Consenso 2015. SEGO (Sociedad Española de Ginecologia y Obstetricia)

[3] Lindqvist PG, Molin J. Does antenatal identification of small-for-gestational age fetuses significantly improve their outcome? Ultrasound in Obstetrics & Gynecology. 2005; **25**:258-264

[4] Richardus JH, Graafmans WC, Verloove-Vanhorick SP, Mackenbach JP, EuroNatal International Audit Panel, EuroNatal Working Group. Differences in perinatal mortality and suboptimal care between 10 European regions: Results of an international audit. BJOG. 2003;**110**:97-105

[5] de Onis M, Garza C, Onyango AW, Martorell R. WHO child growth standards. Acta Paediatrica Suppl. 2006;**450**:1-101

[6] Baschat AA. Doppler application in the delivery timing of the preterm growth-restricted fetuses: Another step in the right direction. Ultrasound in Obstetrics & Gynecology. 2004;**23**:111-118

[7] Hadlock FP, Harrist RB, Sharman RS, Deter RL, Park SK. Estimation of fetal weight with the use of head, body, and femur measurements—A prospective study. American Journal of Obstetrics and Gynecology. 1985;**151**(3):333

[8] Hutcheon JA, Zhang X, Cnattingius S, Kramer MS, Platt RW. Customised birthweight percentiles: Does adjusting for maternal characteristics matter? BJOG. 2008;**115**:1397-1404

[9] Papageorghiou AT, Ohuma EO, Altman DG, Todros T, Cheikh Ismail L, Lambert A, et al. International standards for fetal growth based on serial ultrasound measurements: The fetal growth longitudinal study of the INTERGROWTH-21st project. Lancet. 2014 Sep 6;**384**(9946):869-879

[10] Villar J, Papageorghiou AT, Pang R, Ohuma EO, Cheikh Ismail L, Barros FC, et al. The likeness of fetal growth and newborn size across non-isolated populations in the

INTERGROWTH—21st project: The fetal growth longitudinal study and newborn cross-sectional study. Lancet Diabetes & Endocrinology. 2014 Oct;**2**(10):781-792. Published online July 7

[11] Clausson B, Gardosi J, Francis A, Cnattingius S. Perinatal outcome in SGA births defined by customised versus population-based birthweight standards. BJOG. 2001;**108**:830-834

[12] Baschat AA, Gembruch U. The cerebroplacental Doppler ratio revisited. Ultrasound in Obstetrics & Gynecology. 2003;**21**(2):124-127

[13] Severi FM, Bocchi C, Visentin A, Falco P, Cobellis L, Florio P, et al. Uterine and fetal cerebral Doppler predict the outcome of third-trimester small-for-gestational age fetuses with normal umbilical artery Doppler. Ultrasound in Obstetrics & Gynecology. 2002;**19**(3):225-228

[14] Savchev S, Figueras F, Cruz-Martinez R, Illa M, Botet F, Gratacos E. Estimated weight centile as a predictor of perinatal outcome in small-for-gestational-age pregnancies with normal fetal and maternal Doppler indices. Ultrasound in Obstetrics & Gynecology. 2012;**39**(3):299-303

[15] Figueras F, Gomez L, Eixarch E, Paules C, Mazarico E, Perez M, et al. Defectos del crecimiento fetal. Barcelona: Fetal Medicine Barcelona; 2019. Available from: https://medicinafetalbarcelona.org/protocolos/es/patologia-fetal/defectos-del-crecimiento-fetal.html

[16] Turan OM, Turan S, Gungor S, Berg C, Moyano D, Gembruch U, et al. Progression of Doppler abnormalities in intrauterine growth restriction. Ultrasound in Obstetrics & Gynecology. 2008;**32**(2):160-167

[17] Crovetto F, Crispi F, Scazzocchio E, Mercade I, Meler E, Figueras F, et al. Performance of first trimester integrated screening for early and late small for gestational age newborns. Ultrasound in Obstetrics & Gynecology. 2014 Jan;**43**(1):34-40

[18] Baschat AA, Cosmi E, Bilardo CM, Wolf H, Berg C, Rigano S, et al. Predictors of neonatal outcome in early-onset placental dysfunction. Obstetrics & Gynecology. 2007;**109**(2 Pt 1): 253-261

[19] Hecher K, Bilardo CM, Stigter RH, Ville Y, Hackelöer BJ, Kok HJ, et al. Monitoring of fetuses with intrauterine growth restriction: A longitudinal study. Ultrasound in Obstetrics & Gynecology. 2001;**18**(6):564-570

[20] Oros D, Figueras F, Cruz-Martinez R, Meler E, Munmany M, Gratacos E. Longitudinal changes in uterine, umbilical and fetal cerebral Doppler indices in late-onset small-for-gestational age fetuses. Ultrasound in Obstetrics & Gynecology. 2011;**37**(2):191-195

[21] Gardosi J, Madurasinghe V, Williams M, Malik A, Francis A. Maternal and fetal risk factors for stillbirth: Population based study. BMJ. 2013;**346**:f108

[22] Kady S, Gardosi J. Perinatal mortality and fetal growth restriction. Best Practice & Research: Clinical Obstetrics & Gynaecology. 2004;**18**(3):397-410

[23] Figueras F, Eixarch E, Meler E, Iraola A, Figueras J, Puerto B, et al. Small-for-gestational-age fetuses with normal umbilical artery Doppler have suboptimal perinatal and

neurodevelopmental outcome. European Journal of Obstetrics & Gynecology and Reproductive Biology. 2008;**136**(1):34-38

[24] Larroque B, Bertrais S, Czernichow P, Léger J. School difficulties in 20-year-olds who were born small for gestational age at term in a regional cohort study. Pediatrics. 2001;**108**(1):111-115

[25] Crispi F, Bijnens B, Figueras F, Bartrons J, Eixarch E, Le Noble F, et al. Fetal growth restriction results in remodeled and less efficient hearts in children. Circulation. 2010;**121**(22):2427-36.19

[26] Van Vliet EO et al. Placental pathology and long-term neurodevelopment of very preterm infants. American Journal of Obstetrics and Gynecology. 2012;**206**(6):489.e1-7

[27] Chan PY, Morris JM, Leslie GI, Kelly PJ, Gallery ED. The long-term effects of prematurity and intrauterine growth restriction on cardiovascular, renal, and metabolic function. International Journal Of Pediatrics. 2010;**2010**:280402

[28] Spinillo A, Gardella B, Bariselli S, Alfei A, Silini E, Dal BB. Placental histopathological correlates of umbilical artery Doppler velocimetry in pregnancies complicated by fetal growth restriction. Prenatal Diagnosis. 2012;**32**(13):1263-1272

[29] Llurba E, Turan O, Kasdaglis T, Harman CR, Baschat AA. Emergence of late-onset placental dysfunction: Relationship to the change in uterine artery blood flow resistance between the first and third trimesters. American Journal of Perinatology. 2013;**30**(6):505-512

[30] Lobmaier SM, Figueras F, Mercade I, Perello M, Peguero A, Crovetto F, et al. Angiogenic factors versus Doppler follow up in the prediction of adverse outcome among late pregnancy small-for- gestational-age fetuses. Ultrasound in Obstetrics & Gynecology. 2014;**43**(5):533-540

[31] Enders G, Daiminger A, Bäder U, Exler S, Enders M. Intrauterine transmission and clinical outcome of 248 pregnancies with primary cytomegalovirus infection in relation to gestational age. Journal of Clinical Virology. 2011 Nov;**52**(3):244-246

[32] Higa K, Dan K, Manabe H. Varicella-zoster virus infections during pregnancy: Hypothesis concerning the mechanisms of congenital malformations. Obstetrics & Gynecology. 1987;**69**:214-222

[33] Adams Waldorf KM, McAdams RM. Influence of infection during pregnancy on fetal development. Reproduction. 2013;**146**:R151-R162

[34] Brocklehurst P, French R. The association between maternal HIV infection and perinatal outcome: A systematic review of the literature and meta-analysis. British Journal of Obstetrics and Gynaecology. 1998;**105**(8):836-848

[35] Suy A, Martinez E, Coll O, Lonca M, Palacio M, de Lazzari E, et al. Increased risk of pre- eclampsia and fetal death in HIV-infected pregnant women receiving highly active antiretroviral therapy. AIDS. 2006 Jan 2;**20**(1):59-66

[36] Lopez M, Palacio M, Goncé A, Hernàndez S, Barranco FJ, García L, et al. Risk of intrauterine growth restriction among HIV-infected pregnant women: A cohort study. European Journal of Clinical Microbiology & Infectious Diseases. 2015;**34**:223-230

[37] Conroy AL, Silver KL, Zhong K, Rennie M, Ward P, Sarma JV, et al. Complement activation and the resulting placental vascular insufficiency drives fetal growth restriction associated with placental malaria. Cell Host & Microbe. 2013;**13**:215-226

[38] Snijders RJ, Sherrod C, Gosden CM, Nicolaides KH. Fetal growth retardation: Associated malformations and chromosomal abnormalities. American Journal of Obstetrics and Gynecology. 1993;**168**:547

[39] Figueras F, Meler E, Eixarch E, Francis A, Coll O, Gratacos E, et al. Association of smoking during pregnancy and fetal growth restriction: Subgroups of higher susceptibility. European Journal of Obstetrics & Gynecology and Reproductive Biology. 2008;**138**:171-175

[40] Cruz-Martínez R, Figueras F, Hernandez-Andrade E, Oros D, Gratacos E. Fetal brain Doppler to predict cesarean delivery for nonreassuring fetal status in term small-for-gestational-age fetuses. Obstetrics & Gynecology. 2011;**117**(3):618-626

[41] Gramellini D et al. Cerebral-umbilical Doppler ratio as a predictor of adverse perinatal outcome. Obstetrics & Gynecology. 1992;**79**(3):416-420

[42] Schwarze A, Gembruch U, Krapp M, Katalinic A, Germer U, Axt-Fliedner R. Qualitative venous Doppler flow waveform analysis in preterm intrauterine growth-restricted fetuses with ARED flow in the umbilical artery-correlation with short-term outcome. Ultrasound in Obstetrics & Gynecology. 2005;**25**(6):573-579

[43] Cruz-Lemini M, Crispi F, Van Mieghem T, Pedraza D, Cruz-Martínez R, Acosta-Rojas R, et al. Risk of perinatal death in early-onset intrauterine growth restriction according to gestational age and cardiovascular Doppler indices: A multicenter study. Fetal Diagnosis and Therapy Guidelines. 2012;**32**(1-2):116-122

[44] Fouron JC, Skoll A, Sonesson SE, Pfizenmaier M, Jaeggi E, Lessard M. Relationship between flow through the fetal aortic isthmus and cerebral oxygenation during acute placental circulatory insufficiency in ovine fetuses. American Journal of Obstetrics and Gynecology. 1999;**181**(5 Pt 1):1102-1107

[45] Cruz-Martinez R, Figueras F, Hernandez-Andrade E, Oros D, Gratacos E. Changes in myocardial performance index and aortic isthmus and ductus venosus Doppler in term, small-for-gestational age fetuses with normal umbilical artery pulsatility index. Ultrasound in Obstetrics & Gynecology. 2011;**38**(4):400-405

[46] Fouron JC, Gosselin J, Raboisson MJ, Lamoureux J, Tison CA, Fouron C, et al. The relationship between an aortic isthmus blood flow velocity index and the postnatal neurodevelopmental status of fetuses with placental circulatory insufficiency. American Journal of Obstetrics and Gynecology. 2005;**192**(2):497-503

[47] Grivell RM, Alfirevic Z, Gyte GM, Devane D. Antenatal cardiotocography for fetal assessment. The Cochrane Database of Systematic Reviews. 2010;**1**:CD007863

[48] Lalor JG, Fawole B, Alfirevic Z, Devane D. Biophysical profile for fetal assessment in high risk pregnancies. The Cochrane Database of Systematic Reviews. 2008;**1**:CD007529

[49] Hadlock FP, Deter RL, Harrist RB, Park SK. Estimating fetal age: Computer-assisted analysis of multiple fetal growth parameters. Radiology. 1984 Aug;**152**(2):497-501

[50] Hadlock FP, Harrist RB, Sharman RS, Deter RL, Park SK. Estimation of fetal weight with the use of head, body, and femur measurement. A prospective study. AJOG. 1985;**151**:333-337

[51] Kramer MS, Platt R, Yang H, McNamara H, Usher RH. Are all growth restricted newborns created equal(ly)? Pediatrics. 1999;**103**:599-602

[52] Wolfe HM, Gross TL, Sokol RJ. Recurrent small for gestational age birth: Perinatal risks and out- comes. American Journal of Obstetrics and Gynecology. 1987;**157**:288-293

[53] McCowan L, Horgan RP. Risk factors for small for gestational age infants. Best Practice & Research Clinical Obstetrics & Gynaecology. 2009;**23**:779-793

[54] Khoury MJ, Erickson JD, Cordero JF, McCarthy BJ. Congenital malformations and intrauterine growth retardation: A population study. Pediatrics. 1988;**82**:83

[55] Mendez H. Introduction to the study of pre- and postnatal growth in humans: A review. American Journal of Medical Genetics. 1985;**20**:63

[56] Anandakumar C, Chew S, Wong YC, Malarvishy G, Po LU, Ratnam SS. Early asymmetric IUGR and aneuploidy. Journal of Obstetrics and Gynaecology Research. 1996;**22**:365-370

[57] Yakoob MY, Zakaria A, Waqar SN, Zafar S, Wahla AS, Zaidi SK, et al. Does malaria during pregnancy affect the newborn? Journal of Pakistan Medical Association. 2005;**55**:543-546

[58] Say L, Gulmezoglu MA, Hofmeyer JG. Bed rest in hospital for suspected impaired fetal growth. The Cochrane Database of Systematic Reviews. 1996;**1**:CD000034

[59] McCowan LM, Dekker GA, Chan E, Stewart A, Chappell LC, Hunter M, et al. Spontaneous preterm birth and small for gestational age infants in women who stop smoking early in pregnancy: Prospective cohort study. BMJ. 2009;**338**:b1081

[60] Society of Obstetricians and Gynaecologists of Canada. Intrauterine growth restriction: Screening, diagnosis, and management. Journal of Obstetrics and Gynaecology Canada. 2013;**35**(8):741-748

[61] Baschat AA. Neurodevelopment following fetal growth restriction and its relationship with antepartum parameters of placental dysfunction. Ultrasound in Obstetrics & Gynecology. 2011 May;**37**(5):501-514

[62] Pulver LS, Denney JM, Silver RM, Young PC. Morbidity and discharge timing of late preterm new-borns. Clinical Pediatrics (Phila). 2010 Nov;**49**(11):1061-1067

[63] Nicolaides KH, Bilardo CM, Soothill PW, et al. Absence of end diastolic frequencies in umbilical artery: A sign of fetal hypoxia and acidosis. BMJ. 1988 Oct 22;**297**(6655):1026-1027

[64] Valcamonico A, Danti L, Frusca T, et al. Absent end-diastolic velocity in umbilical artery: Risk of neonatal morbidity and brain damage. American Journal of Obstetrics and Gynecology. 1994 Mar;**170**(3):796-801

[65] Society for Maternal-Fetal Medicine Publications Committee, Berkley E, Chauhan SP, Abuhamad A. Doppler assessment of the fetus with intrauterine growth restriction. American Journal of Obstetrics and Gynecology. 2012 Apr;**206**(4):300-308

[66] Jozwiak M, Bloemenkamp KW, Kelly AJ, Mol BW, Irion O, Boulvain M. Mechanical methods for induction of labour. The Cochrane Database of Systematic Reviews. 2012;**14**:3

Chapter 5

The Role of the Human Growth Hormone Gene Family in Pregnancy

Hugo A. Barrera-Saldaña,
Belinda M. Contreras-Garza and
Silvia A. Barrera-Barrera

Additional information is available at the end of the chapter

http://dx.doi.org/10.5772/intechopen.89011

Abstract

A pregnant woman´s body undergoes profound anatomical and physiological changes to accommodate the needs of the maternal-fetal unit required for a successful pregnancy. During normal pregnancy, the placenta produces a variant of human growth hormone as well as a chorionic somatomammotropin hormone. These are the placental members of the human growth hormone gene family and play a crucial role in the regulation of maternal and fetal metabolism, as well as in the growth and development of the fetus. For this reason, the scope of this chapter is to describe the differences of the biochemical and physiological roles of the hormones coded in this locus during pregnancy, the repercussions of their deficiencies, and role in some of the most prevalent pathologies during pregnancy affecting either the mother or the fetus and also to describe how pioneering sequencing of this locus allowed our laboratory to invent the first companion diagnostics test and thus contributed to the dawn of the personalized medicine era.

Keywords: placenta, growth hormone family, HGH physiology, placental variant HGH, chorionic somatomammotropin hormone, hormonal deficiencies, companion diagnostics, personalized medicine

1. Introduction

The first correlation between growth disorders and the pituitary gland occurred at the beginning of the twentieth century. Human growth hormone (HGH) was later identified as the main promoter of postnatal body growth. Its availability as a recombinant drug at the end of

IntechOpen

© 2019 The Author(s). Licensee IntechOpen. This chapter is distributed under the terms of the Creative Commons Attribution License (http://creativecommons.org/licenses/by/3.0), which permits unrestricted use, distribution, and reproduction in any medium, provided the original work is properly cited.

The 1980s sparked many investigations aimed at exploring many alleged roles in adult health and even in longevity. Likewise, the cloning of its gene and the discovery that it belongs to a gene family along with genes for variant or placental HGH (HGH-V) and chorionic somatomammotropin hormone (CSH: previously referred as placental lactogen) accelerated the understanding of the role of this family in human biology and medicine [1]. Today we understand in detail the molecular mechanisms of their functions, either direct or via mediators, and the role they play in many physiological and pathological processes, although other possible but suspected roles remain unknown. One of the most interesting and fascinating functions of this family of hormones is their contribution to fetal health during pregnancy, although, surprisingly, normal pregnancies with total or partial absences of one or both of the placental hormones have been reported.

2. The HGH family: anatomy, physiology, and homeostasis

In humans, the growth hormone (GH) family includes the pituitary HGH (referred as HGH-N), the placental HGH (named HGH-V), and the CSH; along with prolactin (PRL; a more evolutionarily distant relative) they are collectively referred as somatolactogens. By virtue of their similarities, it was proposed that their genes were derived by gene duplication from a common ancestor dating from the first vertebrates [2]. Over time the members of this family became specialized, developing specific functions: HGH-N has been attributed metabolic and

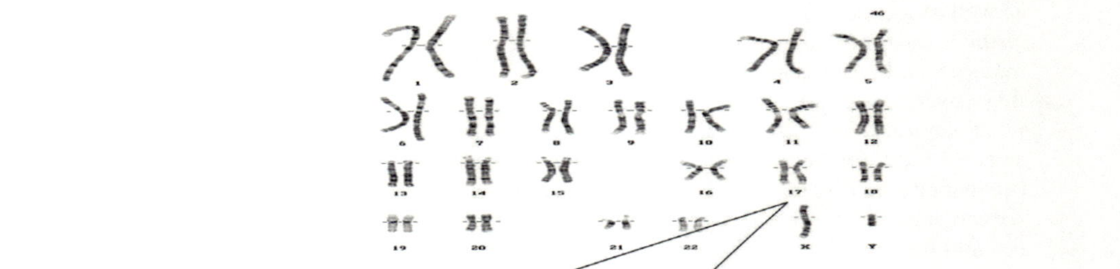

Figure 1. The hGH chapter of the human genome encyclopedia. The *hGH* locus was the first non-highly repetitive DNA element to be localized in the human karyotype. It turned out to harbor the five genes here described. Its sequencing was a world record back in 1988.

somatogenic functions after birth, HGH-V has been attributed metabolic and somatogenic functions during pregnancy, and CSH is considered a lactogenic hormone. PRL is considered a multifunctional hormone [3].

In humans, the *hGH* locus, which includes *hGH* and *hCSH*-type genes, spans approximately 50 kb of band 24.2 at the long arm of chromosome 17. PRL is coded by a single gene that is located on chromosome 6 [4, 5]. The locus′ five genes are arranged in tandem, all in same orientations, and exhibit very high sequence and organizational similarities. At the 5′-end of the locus is the *hGH-N* gene, followed by the pseudogene *hCSH-L*, then *hCSH-1*, next *hGH-V*, and CSH-2 in the end [5] (**Figure 1**).

While the *hGH-N* gene is expressed in the pituitary and yields at least two isoforms (22 and 20 kilo Daltons), the rest do so in the placenta and are responsible: one (*hGH-V*) of the placental variant of HGH or HGH-V and two (*hCSH-1* and *hCSH-2*) for a single mature isoform of HCS. The so-called *hCSH-L* is a pseudogene and thus is postulated to contribute no protein [5].

2.1. Human growth hormone (HGH)

HGH can exert metabolic effects either directly or indirectly through, in the latter case, the increase in hepatic production of the insulin-like growth factor 1 (IGF-1). Regarding their direct actions, the administration of HGH has been reported to antagonize the action of insulin, thus producing intolerance to carbohydrates in spite of elevated plasma insulin levels. In contrast, insulin sensitivity increases during the administration of IGF-1, which exerts hypoglycemic effects even with concomitant suppression of insulin secretion. Another important direct metabolic effect of HGH is to increase the mobilization and oxidation of fat and therefore to reduce total body fat; there is no evidence that IGF-1 acts directly on adipose tissue in vivo. The administration of HGH results in the retention of sodium through the stimulation of Na-K-ATPase. It is suggested that part of the effects of HGH on tubular function (e.g., phosphate reabsorption) is mediated through IGF-1 [6].

The administration of HGH increases the circulating levels of IGF-1 through the stimulation of its hepatic synthesis and secretion; it can also improve the synthesis of local IGF-1 in peripheral tissues, where it exerts autocrine or paracrine effects [6]. While HGH increases lipolysis, as a direct effect on the adipocyte, as well as the oxidation of lipids by increasing substrate availability, IGF-1 increases lipid oxidation only when administered chronically, most likely as a result of chronic insulinopenia. These metabolic regulators have been tested in a variety of catabolic conditions in man, and both hormones have been effective in reducing protein loss caused by glucocorticosteroids and in mitigating some of the catabolic effects of severe hypogonadism in men [7].

Another function of IGF-1 is to increase myelination by increasing the number of myelinated axons and the thickness of myelin sheaths. The latter is by mechanisms involving the stimulation of myelin protein gene expression and by increasing the number of oligodendrocytes [8]. For this reason, people with IGF-1 deficiency, caused by a homozygous mutation in the *IGF-1* gene at the 12q22 locus, present, in addition to intra- and extrauterine growth retardation, mental retardation and sensorineural deafness [9].

Some studies have compared the phenotypes of dwarfism manifested in mutant mice lacking the HGH receptor, or IGF-1, or both, and have provided conclusive evidence that HGH and IGF-1 promote postnatal growth, both by independent and by common functions, given that the delay in the growth of double nullizygotes HGHR/IGF-1 is more severe than that observed with any of the mutant classes separately [10].

2.1.1. Physiological regulation

2.1.1.1. Somatomedins

The insulin-like growth factors, IGF-1 and -2, share structural and functional similarities with insulin. Together with insulin, they make up a family of phylogenetically conserved molecules important in the regulation of both growth and metabolism. IGF-1 and IGF-2 (constitute a small proportion of the total IGFs present in plasma) function predominantly as growth regulators. While it is true that the liver is the source of most (75%) of plasma IGF-1, it is also synthesized by multiple mesenchymal cell types [11]. As a result, there are two main mechanisms of IGF-1 regulation: (1) The IGF-1 that is synthesized in the liver and secreted to the blood is under the control of HGH, and (2) autocrine/paracrine IGF-1 synthesized in peripheral tissues, such as bone, is controlled by HGH and by factors that are secreted locally by the surrounding cell types.

IGF-1 exerts its effects through the activation of the IGF-1 receptor. This receptor is present in multiple types of cells and tissues, which probably explains its ability to stimulate balanced and symmetric growth [12].

2.1.1.2. HGHRH

The role of a GH-releasing hormone (GHRH) in the regulation of HGH secretion has been recognized since the late 1950s, based on several lines of evidence that postulated its existence. These lines of evidence include that the interruption of the connection between the hypothalamus and the pituitary gland leads to a decrease in HGH secretion; that the electrical stimulation of the ventromedial nucleus and the basal hypothalamus stimulates the secretion of HGH; and that hypothalamic crude extracts stimulate the release of HGH from anterior pituitaries in culture [13]. The cell surface receptor for HGHRH (HGHRH-R) has been incompletely characterized. More is known about the post-receptor events triggered by HGHRH. The binding of HGHRH to its receptor stimulates the formation of cyclic AMP, which stimulates an AMPc-dependent protein kinase located in the secretory granules of the pituitary gland, which increases exocytosis of granules and causes the acute release of preformed HGH [13]. HGHRH not only stimulates the release but also stimulates the synthesis of HGH. It has been shown that HGHRH can alter the transcription of the *hGH* gene both in vitro and in vivo, with an increase of 2.5 times 30 minutes after the injection of HGHRH [14].

2.1.1.3. Somatostatin

Somatostatin (SST) is one of the oldest peptides in neurobiology. It was originally discovered in 1972 as part of the hormone-releasing family because of its property to inhibit the secretion of

HGH in monolayers of pituitary cells in vitro. Despite its well-known neuroendocrine effects, it was quickly shown to inhibit a series of endocrine and exocrine secretions along the neural-gut axis including, for example, pancreatic insulin and glucagon or myenteric acid secretions [15].

SST is a cyclic tetradecapeptide synthesized in the hypothalamus, from where it is transported to the anterior pituitary gland where it is responsible for the pulsatile release of HGH and for inhibiting tonically the secretion of HGH and TSH. Several loops of internal feedback, sleep, exercise, and chemical agents control and influence the release of SST [16]. SST acts through six separate surface receptors (SSTR-1, SSTR-1-2A, SSTR-1-2B, SSTR-1-3, SSTR-1-4, SSTR-1-5), members of the family of G protein-coupled receptors, characterized by seven transmembrane-helical domains, creating three intra- and extracellular loops. The binding of the receptor and the ligand (SST/SSTR) results in specific cellular activities for each receptor, or combinations of receptors, and their cellular/tissue localization, although it is known that the common effect is a reduction in cyclic adenosine monophosphate (cAMP) and Ca^{++} with activation of protein phosphatases [16].

3.1.1.4. Other important elements of the pathway

There are many elements whose correct functioning is necessary for the hormonal system of the HGH family to work properly; among the most important of these, we have the transcription factor Pit-l, a member of a POU-domain family of binding factors of DNA; it is a specific pituitary factor that binds to and activates the promoters of both *hGH* and *hPRL* genes. It has also been speculated that Pit-I could play a critical role in the ontogeny of HGH, PRL, and thyroid-stimulating hormone (TSH) producing cells [17].

Another no less important element is prophet of Pit-1 (PROP-1), which is a transcription factor capable of binding to the sites in an early promoter of the *PIT-1* gene and regulating its expression, which is necessary for the development of the pituitary gland and the expression of the hormone [18]. Mutations in this gene have been associated with a combined pituitary hormone deficiency, as well as deficiencies in luteinizing hormone, follicle-stimulating hormone, HGH, PRL, and thyroid-stimulating hormone [18].

2.2. The growth hormone receptor (GHR)

The cloning of the HGH receptor (HGHR) gene in 1987 opened the door for the study of HGH signaling at the molecular level. Its mRNA encodes a protein of 638 amino acids (aa) with single extracellular, transmembrane, and cytoplasmic domains [19]. HGHR belongs to the transmembrane superfamily of proteins that includes the PRL receptor (PRLR) and a number of cytokine receptors [20].

The determination of the structure of HGH bound to the extracellular domain of HGHR has led to the model where a single molecule of HGH binds to two molecules of HGHR. This binding of HGH leading to the HGHR (2)-HGH complex is thought to be sequential. The initial step is the binding of HGH to a high-affinity HGHR monomer, whereby a different face of HGH is contacted by a second HGHR monomer, stabilizing the HGHR dimer. This binding of HGH to its receptor dimer is thought to be an initial and crucial event in the HGH signaling [19]. Subsequent to this, a conformational change in the extracellular domain of the receptor is important for signaling. At present, virtually nothing is known about the structure of the cytoplasmic domain of the HGHR; a clue to the mystery of the signaling mechanism came with the discovery that HGH promotes the tyrosine phosphorylation of receptors and other cellular proteins. The current working model of the signal transduction of HGH action is that its binding to two HGHR monomers increases the affinity of each receptor for JAK2. The dimerization brings two JAK2 molecules in proximity so that each JAK2 can phosphorylate the activation tyrosine of the other JAK2 molecule, blocking it in an active conformation. This allows the activated JAK2 to phosphorylate itself and the cytoplasmic domain of the HGHR in the tyrosine residues, in order to activate the signaling pathway required for the specific function of the HGH that needs to develop: regulation of gene transcription, metabolic actions, etc. [19].

2.3. The IGF receptor

The components of the IGF system include IGFs (IGF-1 and IGF-2), IGF type 1 (IGF-1R), and type 2 (IGF-2R) receptors, a family of six secreted IGF binding proteins (IGFBP) and IGFBP proteases [21]. The two IGF receptors are structurally and functionally related. The signaling of the IGF ligand is mediated by IGF-1R, which is a transmembrane glycoprotein with tyrosine kinase activity. IGF-2R is a single-chain protein with no kinase activity. IGF-1R binds to IGF-1 with up to 20 times higher affinity than with IGF-2, while IGF-2R binds strongly to IGF-2 but hardly recognizes IGF- 1. The genes for IGF2 and IGF2R have imprinting, expressing themselves in a monoallelic way depending on the parental origin [21].

IGF-1R is activated by two ligands, IGF-1 and IGF-2, and by insulin at supraphysiological concentrations [22]. After the binding of IGF-1 to its receptor, it undergoes a conformational

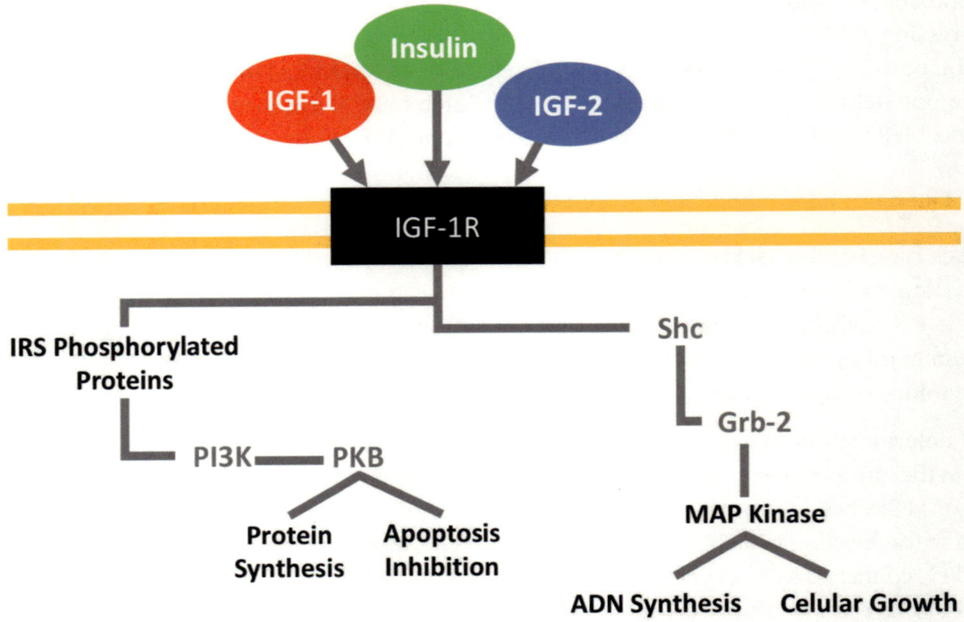

Figure 2. Molecular mechanism of IGF-1R. The signal transduction elicited by insulin and insulin-like growth factors is depicted.

change that unleashes its tyrosine activity kinase (TK). This autophosphorylates tyrosines which act as coupling sites for Shc (a signaling adaptor protein) and IRS-1 or IRS-2 signaling proteins. The IRS proteins are phosphorylated by the TK activity of the receptor and then binds to the p85 subunit of phosphatidylinositol 3-kinase (PI3K), which is the type A regulatory/subunit of the isoforms of class 1 of the PI3K, leading to the activation of protein kinase B (PKB) and the stimulation of protein synthesis, as well as the inhibition of apoptosis. The Shc signaling protein is also phosphorylated, which allows it to bind to growth factor receptor-bound protein 2 (Grb-2), leading to the activation of MAP kinase and the stimulation of DNA synthesis and cell growth (**Figure 2**).

The critical importance of this receptor for normal development and physiology is underlined by neonatal lethality as a result of its complete absence. Conversely, IGF-2R, also called mannose-6-phosphate receptor independent of cations, is less important for growth stimulation but is important for the regulation of IGF-1 and IGF-2 activities, both by sequestration of hormones, as by promoting their degradation [23].

IGF-2 is a key regulator of cell growth, survival, migration, and differentiation. Its fundamental role in these processes requires strict regulation, both of expression and activity. The IGF-1R mediates the actions of IGF-2, and a family of six high-affinity binding proteins of IGF (IGFBP-1 to IGFBP-6) regulates the circulating half-life of IGF-2 and its availability to bind to IGF-1R. In addition, IGF2-R modulates circulating and tissue levels of IGF-2, directing it to lysosomes for degradation [23].

An example of the growth regulation function of IGF-2 is the Beckwith-Wiedemann syndrome (BWS), which is a pediatric overgrowth disorder with predisposition to form embryonic tumors. Individuals with BWS can grow at a higher rate during the second half of pregnancy and in the first years of life [24]. BWS results from alterations in the imprint control region 1 (ICR1), either by deletion or by DNA methylation. The ICR1 region controls the genomic imprint of the *H19* gene, a gene that, unlike many others, does not code for a protein but rather a noncoding RNA molecule whose function is unknown, although it is suspected that it acts as a suppressor of the tumor and of the *IGF-2* gene, which has already been mentioned previously. This anomaly alters the regulation of both genes; specifically, it leads to a loss of the activity of the *H19* gene and an increase in the activity of the *IGF-2* gene in many tissues [25].

3. HGH and IGF-1 during pregnancy

The pregnant woman undergoes profound anatomic and physiologic changes in almost every organ system. These adaptations to the pregnant state begin just after conception and evolve through delivery, after which they almost completely revert to the nonpregnant state over a period of weeks. The purpose of these alterations is to accommodate the needs of the maternal-fetal unit.

During pregnancy, pituitary HGH-N synthesis in the mother is suppressed, and HGH-V starts to be synthesized by the placenta, becoming the predominant HGH in the pregnant women [26]. There is no precise explanation in the literature of the differential actions of HGH-N and HGH-V. It is considered that HGH-V plays an essential role for healthy intrauterine development by increasing the levels of IGF-1, favoring its bioavailability for the fetus, and generating an insulin resistance through its lower lactogenic effects to ensure a contribution of constant glucose.

The evolution of serum HGH-N in pregnant women has been studied with radioimmunoassays (RIA) unreactive to CSH. In such women, serum HGH-N levels progressively decline to undetectable levels during the second half of pregnancy, while HGH-V appears in the circulation at midpregnancy and increases thereafter up to term [27]. HGH-V is secreted by the placenta in a non-pulsatile manner. This continuous secretion appears to have important implications for physiological adjustment to gestation and especially in the control of maternal IGF-1 levels [5]. The "normal" episodic peak activity of HGH-V in first-trimester pregnant women is dramatically changed into a continuous very stable secretion during late pregnancy. This change is first observed at 17 weeks of gestation. It is concluded that during the second half of pregnancy, serum measurements of HGH reflect a major contribution from a non-episodically secreted placental HGH-V and concomitant suppression of pituitary HGH-N. This specific signal, i.e., a continuous HGH secretion, may be an important regulator of maternal liver metabolism during pregnancy and is directly involved in the insulin resistance of pregnancy [28, 29].

Placental HGH-V is the same length (191 aa) as pituitary HGH-N but contains 13 different aa, is more basic, and possesses one glycosylation site. These small differences are thought to be responsible for the reduced lactogenic and high somatogenic activities of placental HGH-V compared with pituitary HGH-N [5, 30]. In vitro placental HGH-V binds to HGHR with similar affinity than pituitary HGH-N. However, placental HGH-V has considerably lower affinity than pituitary HGH for lactogenic receptors [5]. CSH and PRL increase maternal food intake by induction of central leptin resistance and promotion of maternal beta-cell expansion and insulin production to defend against the development of gestational diabetes mellitus. It is probable that as a result of the lower affinity of placental HGH-V for lactogenic receptors than pituitary HGH-N and the fact that its secretion is not suppressible by high glucose levels, pregnancy is a well-known period of susceptibility for the development of diabetes and other metabolically alterations. HGH-V is equipotent to pituitary HGH-N as a ligand for circulating HGH binding protein and therefore circulates in the maternal circulation as both free and bound HGH-V [5].

3.1. Growth hormone-releasing hormone

HGH releasing hormone (HGHRH) is a 44 aa peptide. Its concentration throughout pregnancy is similar to that in nonpregnant women despite fluctuations in HGH values, which are always higher than in nonpregnant levels [31], thus supporting the idea that HGH values are higher during pregnancy due to the placental secretion of HGH-V not regulated by HGHRH [29].

After delivery, placental HGH-V disappears from maternal serum within an hour. Amniotic fluid contains low HGH concentrations; cord serum contains high HGH levels, but not because of HGH-V (we assumed that the material responsible for the GH immunoreactivity in late pregnancy maternal serum was of placental origin, since it rapidly disappeared after delivery); thus, it appears to be secreted selectively into the maternal compartment [27].

HGH-V does not appear to have a direct effect on fetal growth as it is secreted only in the maternal circulation and is not detected in the fetal blood [5]. Secreted continuously by the placenta, it seems to control the synthesis of maternal IGF-1; indeed, maternal IGF-1 levels are correlated with placental HGH levels [30]. Its continuous secretion by syncytiotrophoblast villous into the maternal compartment may alter maternal metabolism during pregnancy. In the maternal liver and other organs, HGH-V strongly stimulates gluconeogenesis, lipolysis, and anabolism, thereby increasing nutrient availability for the fetoplacental unit [5]. HGH-V acts in vivo as an HGH-N agonist sharing most of its biological properties [27]. HGH-N, which is synthesized by the fetal pituitary gland (levels of which rise to a maximum at mid-gestation) [26], has little or no physiological action on the fetus until the end of pregnancy, because of the lack of functional HGH receptors in fetal tissues.

Growth, prenatal development, and size at birth are normal in animal fetuses of specimens subjected to hypophysectomy and HGH deficiency, including human fetuses with mutant genes for this and their receptors. However, this pattern is not maintained in the postnatal period, in which the individual manifests abnormal development and growth [21]. HGH deficiency does not eliminate the normal increase in IGF-1 induced by pregnancy and does not reduce fetal weight [30]. Unlike IGF-2 levels, the levels of HGH-V do not correlate with birth weight or placental weight [32].

In humans and mice, mutations or specific deletions of the genes for IGFs, IGF1, and IGF2, as well as IGF1R and for its main signaling molecule IRS, lead to a restriction in fetal growth [33]. The targeted inactivation of the mouse gene for IGF-2 results in a 40% reduction in fetal growth, but postnatal growth remains normal so that alterations in development occur exclusively in the prenatal period. On the other hand, the interruption of the *IGF-1* gene leads to a similar decrease in fetal growth than the alteration of the *IGF-2* gene, but it is also characterized by the lack of persistent postnatal growth [34]. Most surprising, however, are the phenotypic consequences of the deletion of the gene for the IGF-1 receptor (IGF-1R), which as described above, is a transmembrane tyrosine kinase that mediates the growth promotion actions of both IGFs. Mice with this suppression have a birth weight that is only 45% of normal and usually die in a matter of hours after birth due to respiratory failure as a result of muscle hypoplasia [34].

3.2. Growth hormone replacement therapy during pregnancy

A retrospective study of 25 women with HGH-N deficiency (HGHD), who underwent pregnancy without HGH replacement therapy (HGHRT), concluded that unsubstituted HGHD during pregnancy is not detrimental to the fetus [35]. Another publication described four HGHD women who stopped HGHRT immediately after confirmation of pregnancy and remained off treatment throughout the pregnancy while having no pregnancy complications and gave birth to healthy babies of normal height and weight [36]. In a case report, physiologic HGHRT until there was evidence of sufficient HGH-V production also led to normal pregnancy and a healthy fetus [37]. This regimen of maintaining HGHRT during the first trimester, gradually decreasing it during the second trimester, and discontinuing it during the third trimester was reported to lead to successful outcomes in 12 pregnancies [38]. In addition, replacement with HGH-N during pregnancy did not suppress the physiologic increase in HGH-V [32].

Author	Pregnancy outcome	Product outcome	Hormone level/ molecular characterization
Alexander *et al.*	Normal pregnancy with spontaneous labor at 39 weeks	Normal female infant; weighted 3300 g	CSH level < 0.006 mg/l. No molecular analysis
Barbieri *et al.*	Normal pregnancy	Normal product	CSH absent, confirmed by immunoperoxidase technique
Borody and Carlton	Normal pregnancy (second pregnancy)	Healthy female infant	CSH deficiency. No molecular analysis
Bradford and Hargreaves	Normal pregnancy (primigravida)	Term male infant, weighing 3420 g	CSH < 2.0 mg/l. No molecular analysis
Geade *et al.*	Normal pregnancy (primigravida). Medical induction of labor at term	Male infant weighing 3740 g	CSH < 1 mg/l. No molecular analysis
Giampietro *et al.*	Normal pregnancy (second pregnancy) with Cesarean section at 39th week for alterations in fetal heart rate	Healthy male infant, weighing 3060 g, 51 cm tall, cranial circumference of 34 cm.	CSH levels between 0.8 and 1.4 μg/ml. No molecular analysis
Hubert *et al.*	Normal pregnancy	Normal product	CSH levels low. Messenger RNA coding for CSH at low abundance
Moshirpur *et al.*	Normal pregnancy	Healthy male infant	CSH <1 μg/ml. No molecular analysis
Nielsen *et al.*	Normal pregnancy (fourth pregnancy). Spontaneous delivery	Healthy male infant, weighing 3000 g, 53 cm tall	CSH <0.025 mg/L. No molecular analysis
Parks *et al.*	Normal pregnancy, with spontaneous delivery at 38 weeks of gestation	Healthy female infant, weighing 2650 g, 49 cm tall	Isolated partial deficiency of CSH (peak CSH levels 1.1 μg/ml). Characterized by restriction endonucleases analysis (heterozygosity for two different deletions involving *hCSH* genes; the paternal *hGH* locus lacked the *hCS-1*, *hGH-V*, and *hCS-2* genes, while the maternal only the *hCS-1* gene)
Sideri *et al.*	Normal pregnancy (third pregnancy) with slight fetal growth impairment. Spontaneous labor at 38 weeks of gestation	Healthy female infant weighting 2600 g (a value just below the 10th centile by normal Italian standards)	No CSH could be measured by RIA. PRL and HGH levels were within the normal limits (137 and 14 ng/ml), and an oral glucose tolerance test at 30 weeks was normal
Simon *et al.*	Two normal pregnancies.	Patient 1: Healthy female infant, weighing 3640 g Patient 2: Healthy female infant, weighing 3250 g	DNA was investigated for the integrity of the *hGH* gene cluster by Southern blotting and hybridization with an *hCSH* cDNA probe. Patient 1 was found to be homozygous for a deletion involving *hCSH-1*, *hGH-V*, and *hCSH-2*. Patient 2 was a double heterozygote, with one chromosome bearing the same deletion as that of patient 1, while in the other, only the *hCSH-1* gene was missing

Table 1. Comparison of reported pregnancy cases with absence of CSH or very low concentrations in maternal plasma [40–51].

A study describing pregnancies in a large group of patients (173 pregnancies in 144 women with HGHD) in 15 countries using the Pfizer International Metabolic Database (KIMS) demonstrates that most patients conceived while receiving HGHRT. Details of HGHRT during pregnancy were reported in 170 out of 173 pregnancies. HGHRT was stopped at the beginning of the pregnancy (or had already been stopped before conception) in 81 cases (46.7%), partially continued in 42 pregnancies (24.7%), and continued throughout the entire pregnancy in 47 pregnancies (27.6%). The practice of partially continuing HGHRT during pregnancy and stopping it at the end of the second trimester was observed in nearly half of the countries but was more prevalent in Sweden (67% of all pregnancies in that country) and Denmark (55% of Danish pregnancies). Most physicians reported making their decisions about whether to continue HGHRT in agreement with the patient's wish. Outcome data were available for 139 pregnancies (80.3% of cases). In four cases the pregnancy was electively terminated (in three cases because of the patient's wish, in one case because of the doctor's advice given several concomitant diseases and the resulting need for multiple medications); these cases were excluded from further analysis. Live birth was observed in 107 pregnancies (79% of all known cases), with a total of 118 babies born. No congenital malformations were reported. No live births were reported in 28 pregnancies, including two extrauterine pregnancies, one blighted ovum (non-evolutive pregnancy), one malformation (severe cystic hygroma in ultrasound, which determined pregnancy termination in the second trimester), one stillbirth, and 23 non-elective abortions. Patients who partially or fully continued HGHRT during the pregnancy did not report any miscarriages happening after the first trimester of the pregnancy [39].

There are few reported cases in the literature of pregnancies with the absence of CSH or very low concentrations in maternal plasma throughout pregnancy, most of them progressing normally and resulting in delivery of normal babies, but only in a few cases have had the genetic background examined in detail using molecular analysis (**Table 1**).

4. Role of hGH locus in pioneering personalized medicine

Biotechnology has not only been a great ally in the diagnosis of diseases but has become part of the treatment, in the specific case of HGH through the development of HGH and CSH recombinant versions. With this, the era of personalized medicine begins, which refers to the design and application of prevention, diagnosis, and treatment strategies better adapted to the genetic-molecular specificities of each patient and each disease. That is, instead of all patients being treated in a similar way, more and more, the treatments will be adapted to groups of selected patients defined by molecular markers (**Figure 3**) [52].

The first step of this personalized medicine is to know the molecular substrate of the diseases that we face. The invention of the first companion diagnostic test was to screen for deletions in the *HGH* locus in search of explaining the failure of HGHRT due to immune rejection of the biosynthetic version of HGH. Using bioinformatics methods, our laboratory analyzed the *hGH* and *hCSH* genes. On the basis of the high sequence similarity displayed by these genes, we designed an ingenious strategy based on restriction enzyme characterizations that allow differentiating each gene's transcriptional unit. To simplify the gene analyses, gene regions

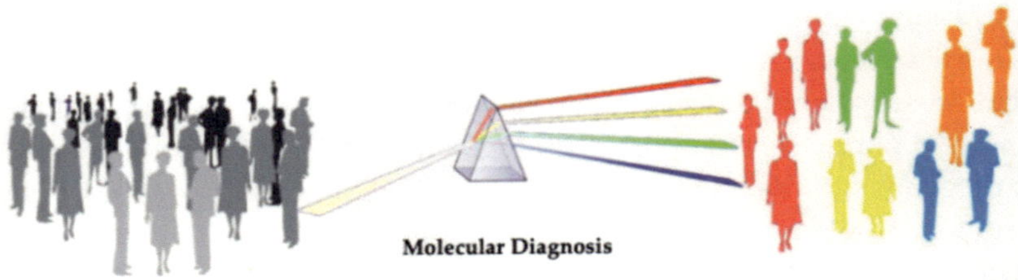

Figure 3. Stratification of patients by molecular diagnosis. Patients apparently with the same disease usually have genetic and thus physiological differences that influence their disease prognosis and prediction.

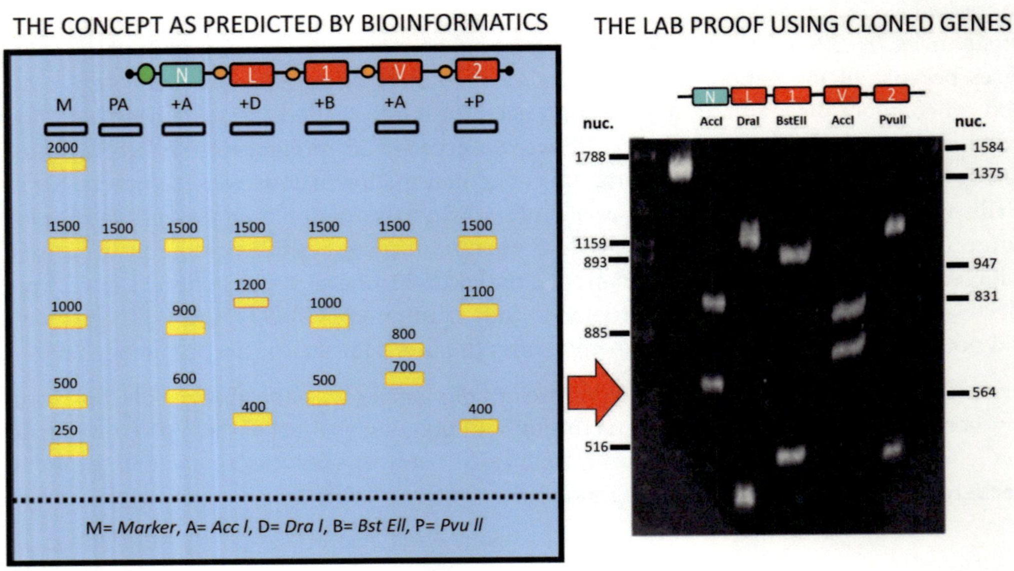

Figure 4. Diagnostic test for the *hGH* locus. Bioinformatics prediction and confirmation in the laboratory of the PCR + restriction enzymes test to differentiate each of the five genes constituents of the *hGH* locus. The gene-specific digestion patterns predicted *in silico* when amplifying all genes by a simple consensus primers PCR and then subjecting the pentagenic amplicon to "diagnostic" restriction enzymes were confirmed using cloned versions of all the gene members of this gene family.

of highest similarities were identified by means of the GENEALIGN program [53, 54]. This analysis resulted in the synthesis of a pair of consensus oligonucleotides complementary to the extremes of the five genes, allowing their simultaneous amplification by PCR. We chose as useful for this purpose what we call diagnostic restriction endonucleases: *Acc* I for *hGH-N* (0.9 and 0.6 kb) and *hGH-V* (0.8 and 0.7 kb), *Dra* I for *hCSH-L* (1.2 and 0.3 kb), *Bst* EII for *hCSH-1* (1.0 and 0.5 kb), and *Pvu* II for *hCSH-2* (1.1 and 0.4 kb) [53].

To test our bioinformatics-predicted test, we then used recombinant plasmids carrying the genes of the locus to confirm the presence of the restriction site for the chosen diagnostic endonuclease for each gene. Amplifications and digestion of each gene-carrying plasmid were performed. The digested PCR products were separated by 1.5% agarose gel electrophoresis. In all cases, we obtained the expected results (**Figure 4**). Fragments corresponding to the *hGH-N* gene (0.9 and 0.6 kb) and *hGH-V* gene (0.8 and 0.7 kb) were seen when *Acc* I was used to digest the amplified products of plasmids containing *hGH-N* and *hGH-V* genes, respectively. Likewise, fragments of 1.2 and 0.3 kb were generated with *Dra* I upon digestion of the PCR product of recombinant plasmid carrying the *hCSH-L* gene. The digestion of the amplified product derived from the *hCSH-1* gene-carrying plasmid with *Bst* EII gave bands of 1.0 and 0.5 kb. Finally, the digestion with *Pvu* II of the amplified product of the cloned gene *hCSH-2* gave bands of 1.1 and 0.4 kb. No unexplained additional fragments were observed in both amplifications and cutting reactions, which reflects the specificity of the PCR and of the cuts with the chosen so-called diagnostic restriction endonucleases [53].

4.1. Application of the diagnostic test

4.1.1. *A case of absence of CSH and HGH-V*

In a pregnancy reported without HCS and HGH-V production, which was complicated by severe growth retardation of the fetus and mild preeclampsia and cardiotocogram abnormalities, the patient was given betamethasone, and Cesarean section was performed in week 35. A male baby was delivered with an Apgar score of 7/1, 10/5 and umbilical artery pH of 7.3, weight was 1270 g, and he measured 40 cm (the 10th percentile for weight for Danish male reference material at this gestational age is 2100 grams). Placenta weight was 250 g and was macroscopically normal. The umbilical cord contained only one artery. A thorough examination of the baby by a neonatologist revealed no physical abnormalities. The boy thrived; the only problem being a tendency to low blood sugar the first days, the lowest being 1.2 mM. He was discharged 26 days after delivery. Pediatric examination at discharge and 6 months later revealed no malformations or other problems [54].

Using the PCR method described before, the genes at the *hGH* multigene family were investigated in DNA isolated from the placenta of this case. We found that the placenta, and thus the baby, had two different DNA deletions along the 3′ half of the gene cluster, both of which eliminated the two active *hCSH* genes (*hCSH-1* and *hCSH-2*) and the placental *hGH* gene (*hGH-V*). The locus retained the pituitary *hGH-N* gene as well as the placental *hCSH-L* pseudogene (see **Figure 5**). The absence of CSH in this patient was caused by deletion of both copies in each chromosome of the active *hCSH* genes (*hCSH-1* and *hCSH-2*) in the placenta and, thus, in the child's genome. Both parents were heterozygous for the gene's deletion, lacking one copy of the three 3′ cluster genes: *hCSH-1*, *hGH-V*, and *hCSH-2*. In the first instance, the baby appeared to be a homozygote for deletion including the 3′ end of the *hGH* locus, but the PCR analysis revealed that the baby was, in fact, a double heterozygote for these deletions. Each chromosome lacks a different portion of the 3′ end of the *hGH* locus: one deletion begins between *hCSH-L* and *hCSH-1* genes and the other beginning at the first exon of the *hCSH-1* gene [54]. In the few previous reports where the molecular background for complete absence or very low levels of CSH have been examined [55], the cause has also been the deletion of *hCSH-1*, *hGH-V*, and *hCSH-2* genes or only of the last two genes, and in some cases both types of *hCSH* gene deletion have been found [49].

4.1.2. *Cases of children treated with recombinant HGH to treat their severe growth retardation*

Genomic DNA samples of 10 patients clinically diagnosed with isolated HGH deficiency (IGHD) were analyzed with our new diagnostic method, to establish if the *hGH-N* gene was absent and thus was the causal factor for this condition. Amplification products of all patients

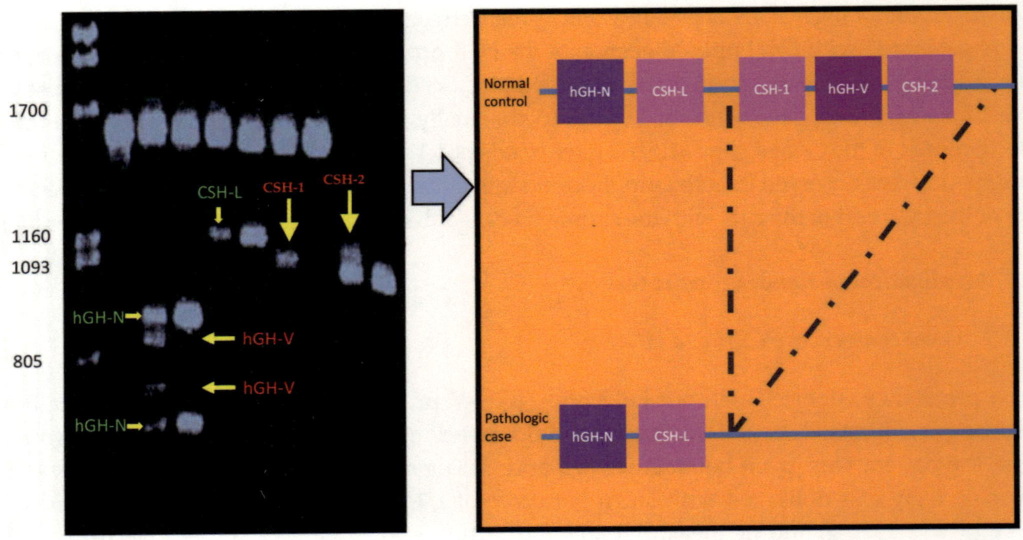

Figure 5. Molecular characterization of a case lacking CSH. Amplification by PCR with our consensus pair of primers capable of amplifying the five genes in the *hGH* locus, followed by digestion with "diagnostic" restriction enzymes, allowed to precise which genes were absent from the genome of the baby in this case of the complete absence of HGH-V and of CSH.

were digested with *Acc* I, which is specific for the *hGH-N* gene (0.9 and 0.6 kb) and for the *hGH-V* gene (0.8 and 0.7 kb) genes. This indicated to us that the former gene was absent in this child and, thus, the cause of this patient's disease, classifying her condition as IGHD type IA. Moreover, the pediatrician confirmed to us that this particular patient was not responding to the HGHRT [53] (**Figure 6**).

4.2. Anti-recombinant growth hormone antibodies

Pituitary HGH has been the preferred treatment for growth retardation in children since its efficacy was first reported 40 years ago. This treatment was discontinued in most countries in 1985 following the deaths from Creutzfeldt-Jakob disease of four patients who received the hormone recovered from cadavers in the period of 1965 through 1975. Application of recombinant (r) DNA technology has made the production of unlimited supplies of proteins possible, including HGH that has important therapeutic uses. But, the immunogenicity of commercially available rHGH is a matter of great concern. The adjuvant effects of unrelated contaminants associated with rHGH by disulfide, ionic and/or hydrophobic links, as well as the changes in the intrinsic primary and secondary structure, may occur during the production and/or recovery of the hormone and lead to potential immunogenicity. The main concern with anti-HGH antibodies could be their ability to neutralize circulating rHGH and inhibiting its growth-promoting effect. In a study evaluating 47 children treated with rHGH for up to 6 months, serum samples were examined for specific antibodies against it by ELISA, resulting in four patients positive for serum antibodies against the hormone [56]. Fortunately, new preparations have shown lower immunogenicity profile with no safety concerns [57].

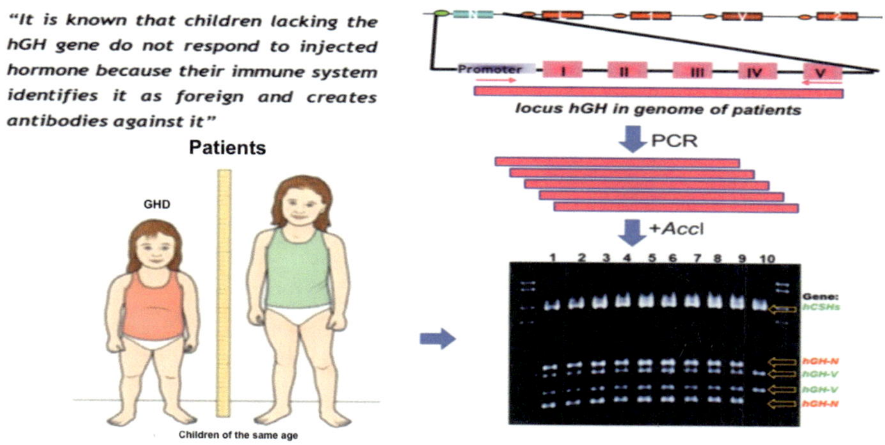

Figure 6. A genetic test to identify HGH-deficient patients that would not respond to replacement therapy from those that would. Bioinformatics analyses of the sequences of the five genes of the *hGH* locus allowed us to design a simple polymerase chain reaction with just one pair of consensus primers to amplify them. Digestion of the mixture of amplicons with *Acc* 1 restriction enzyme should render a ladder of four digestion bands: The first and last bands are digestion products of the gene responsible, in the hypophysis, for the synthesis of HGH (*hGH-N*), while the second and third bands are evidence of the presence of the placental gene counterpart (*hGH-V*) [52].

In a study of four patients with gene defects in the GH axis, the results showed that HGH substitution may be effective at the beginning, but development of HGH-Ab often occurs, resulting in a HGH-resistant state with sequelae similar to GHIS (HG insensitivity syndrome). One patient [58] developed high-affinity and high-avidity blocking of HGH-Ab during the first year of pituitary-derived human GH (pit-GH) treatment. Even plasmapheresis and immune modulating treatment to induce tolerance analogous to previous treatment regimes in hemophiliac patients with blocking antibodies did not result in HGH responsiveness, and HGH-Ab reappeared shortly thereafter [59]. The HGH growth response, even in patients with the identical genetic defect, may differ and is not clearly related to the presence of antibodies [60]. Factors contributing to immune response are complex and cannot be clearly demonstrated. Epidemiology and risk factors of HGH-Ab development have not been studied in depth, but analogous to hemophilia, there are various aspects that might be deduced: On a superior level, immune processes of self–/non-self-discrimination, i.e., the likelihood that antibodies will be formed appears to be influenced by the age at first antigen contact, the HLA haplotype, and other immune response genes. In particular, epitopes giving rise to antibody formation may differ and lead to various effects which are dependent on steric conformation changes or potency of complement activation [61]. Patients with genetic HGH defects who are exposed to exogenous rHGH will therefore generate different amounts of HGH-Ab with different affinities, thus compromising HGH binding to the receptor or HGHBP/HGHR (GH binding protein and GH receptor) dimerization kinetics [62]. In patients with different HGHR mutations, the extent of height deficit varies substantially and may be correlated with the presence or absence of HGHBP in plasma, although clear genotype–phenotype associations do not exist, thus suggesting an influence of additional genes or environmental factors [63–66]. The clinical outcome of treatment with rHGH in patients with IGHD IA is quite variable. The amount and the affinity of GH-Ab modulated by genetic disposition for immune reactions may determine the overall response to HGH therapy [62].

5. Summary

During the prenatal period, the product has a very rapid development, for which it needs an adequate supply of nutrients by the mother. To date, many factors involved in this growth have been described. However, one of the most important without a doubt is the somatogenic and lactogenic hormones (collectively referred to as somatolactogens). Being the intrauterine period essential to define the health of the product throughout its extrauterine life, it is logical to think that there are biological mechanisms in nature that were evolving to assure the nutrient supply through the placenta. Many data point to the fact that HGH-V is one of these biological mechanisms.

During pregnancy, the expression of pituitary HGH is suppressed, and placental HGH becomes the predominant form of HGH in the mother [26]. This change in HGH production indicates that there must be some difference in their functions and surely have implications in the normal evolution of pregnancy. One of these differences is that HGH-V is secreted by the placenta in a non-pulsatile manner. This continuous secretion seems to have important implications in the physiological adjustment to gestation and especially in the control of maternal IGF-1 levels [5].

The lower affinity of HGH-V for the lactogenic receptors and the fact that its secretion is not suppressed by the high levels of blood glucose prevent glucose from being picked up by the mother's tissues and thus being available to the fetus. However, these effects also cause the pregnancy to be a period of susceptibility to the development of diabetes and other metabolic disorders, as is well known. HGH-V does not have a direct effect on fetal growth since it is secreted selectively into the maternal compartment and is not detected in fetal blood [27]. The effect on fetal growth apparently occurs indirectly through the IGF-1 maternal. HGH-V is secreted continuously by the placenta and that seems to control the synthesis of maternal IGF-1. This is supported by the fact that maternal IGF-1 levels are correlated with HGH-V levels. In addition, it binds to the hepatic receptors of HGH with a higher potency than HGH-N [27].

Unlike HGH-N, HGH-V does not increase the transcription of genes from the other components of the IGF system [IGF-2, IGF-2R, IGF-1R, a family of six IGF binding proteins (IGFBPs), and IGFBP proteases]. Therefore, during pregnancy, when HGH-V takes control over HGH-N, there is a greater amount of free IGF-1 available, which may be one of the reasons for the evolutionary divergence of the *hGH* locus for the creation of two GHs that will act in different periods of life.

Besides being the *hGH* locus a wonderful model to investigate gene spatial and temporal expression control, its world-record sequencing and pioneer translation into the first companion diagnostic ever invented, inaugurated the era of personalized medicine.

Acknowledgements

The authors thank Alfredo Ulloa-Aguirre, MD, and Rolando H. González for valuable suggestions and the National Council of Science and Technology (CONACyT) of the Mexican government for support.

Author details

Hugo A. Barrera-Saldaña[1,2]*, Belinda M. Contreras-Garza[3] and Silvia A. Barrera-Barrera[2]

*Address all correspondence to: habarrera@gmail.com

1 Vitagénesis SA, Monterrey, Nuevo León, México

2 Innbiogem SC at National Laboratory for Specialized Services of Research, Development, and Innovation on Chemical and Biotechnological Drugs (LANSEIDI)-CONACyT, Monterrey, Nuevo León, México

3 National Respiratory Diseases Institute, México City, México

References

[1] Lindholm J. Growth hormone: Historical notes. Pituitary. 2006;**9**(1):5-10

[2] Bermea KC, Rodríguez-García A, Tsin A, Barrera-Saldaña HA. Somatolactogens and diabetic retinopathy. Growth Hormone and IGF Research. 2018;**41**:42-47

[3] Goffin V, Shiverick KT, Kelly PA, Martial JA. Sequence-function relationships within the expanding family of prolactin, growth hormone, placental lactogen, and related proteins in mammals. Endocrine Reviews. 1996;**17**(4):385-410

[4] Chen EY, Liao YC, Smith DH, Barrera-Saldaña HA, Gelinas RE, Seeburg PH. The human growth hormone locus: Nucleotide sequence, biology, and evolution. Genomics. 1989;**4**(4):479-497

[5] Lacroix MC, Guibourdenche J, Frendo JL, Muller F, Evain-Brion D. Human placental growth hormone—A review. Placenta. 2002;**23**:S87-S94. DOI: 10.1053/plac.2002.0811

[6] Berneis K, Keller U. Metabolic actions of growth hormone: Direct and indirect. Baillière's Clinical Endocrinology and Metabolism. 1996;**10**(3):337-352

[7] Mauras N, Haymond MW. Are the metabolic effects of GH and IGF-I separable? Growth Hormone and IGF Research. 2005;**15**(1):19-27. DOI: 10.1016/j.ghir.2004.12.003

[8] Ye PING, Carson J, D'Ercole AJ. In vivo actions of insulin-like growth factor-I (IGF-1) on brain myelination: Studies of IGF-1 and IGF binding protein-1 (IGFBP-1) transgenic mice. The Journal of Neuroscience. 1995;**15**(11):7344-7356

[9] Online Mendelian Inheritance in Man, OMIM®. Baltimore, MD: Johns Hopkins University; 2014. MIM#: {608747}: [Accessed: 21 May 2014]. World Wide Web URL: http://omim.org

[10] Lupu F, Terwilliger JD, Lee K, Segre GV, Efstratiadis A. Roles of growth hormone and insulin-like growth factor 1 in mouse postnatal growth. Developmental Biology. 2001;**229**(1):141-162

[11] Murphy LJ. The role of the insulin-like growth factors and their binding proteins in glucose homeostasis. Journal Diabetes Research. 2003;**4**(4):213-224

[12] Werner H, Weinstein D, Bentovl. Similarities and differences between insulin and IGF-1: Structures, receptors, and signaling pathways. Archives of Physiology and Biochemistry. 2008;**114**(1):17-22

[13] Gelato MC, Merriam GR. Growth hormone releasing hormone. Annual Review of Physiology. 1986;**48**(1):569-591

[14] Barinaga M, Yamonoto G, Rivier C, Vale W, Evans R, Rosenfeld MG. Transcriptional regulation of growth hormone gene expression by growth hormone-releasing factor. Nature. 1983;**306**(5938):84-85. DOI: 10.1038/306084a0

[15] Epelbaum J. Somatostatin in the central nervous system: Physiology and pathological modifications. Progress in Neurobiology. 1986;**27**(1):63-100. DOI: 10.1016/0301-0082(86) 90012-2

[16] Barnett P. Somatostatin and somatostatin receptor physiology. Endocrine. 2003;**20**(3):255-264. DOI: 10.1385/endo:20:3:255

[17] Ohta K, Nobukuni Y, Mitsubuchi H, Fujimoto S, Matsuo N, Inagaki H, et al. Mutations in the Pit-1 gene in children with combined pituitary hormone deficiency. Biochemical and Biophysical Research Communications. 1992;**189**(2):851-855

[18] Pruitt KD, Tatusova T, Brown GR, Maglott DR. NCBI reference sequences (RefSeq): Current status, new features and genome annotation policy. Nucleic Acids Research. 2012;**40**(D1):D130-D135

[19] Herrington J, Carter-Su C. Signaling pathways activated by the growth hormone receptor. Trends in Endocrinology and Metabolism. 2001;**12**(6):252-257

[20] Postel-Vinay MC, Kelly PA. Growth hormone receptor signalling. Baillière's Clinical Endocrinology and Metabolism. 1996;**10**(3):323-336

[21] Agrogiannis GD, Sifakis S, Patsouris ES, Konstantinidou AE. Insulin-like growth factors in embryonic and fetal growth and skeletal development (review). Molecular Medicine Reports. 2014;**10**(2):579-584

[22] Baserga R. Customizing the targeting of IGF-1 receptor. Future Oncology. 2009;**5**(1):43-50

[23] Brown J, Jones EY, Forbes BE. Keeping IGF-1I under control: Lessons from the IGF-1I-IGF2R crystal structure. Trends in Biochemical Sciences. 2009;**34**(12):612-619

[24] Weksberg R, Shuman C, Beckwith JB. Beckwith–Wiedemann syndrome. European Journal of Human Genetics. 2010;**18**(1)

[25] IGF2. 2008. Recuperado de http://ghr.nlm.nih.gov/gene/IGF2

[26] Handwerger S, Freemark M. The roles of placental growth hormone and placental lactogen in the regulation of human fetal growth and development. Journal of Pediatric Endocrinology and Metabolism. 2000;**13**(4):343-356

[27] Frankenne F, Closset J, Gomez F, Scippo ML, Smal J, Hennen G. The physiology of growth hormones (GHs) in pregnant women and partial characterization of the placental hGH variant. The Journal of Clinical Endocrinology and Metabolism. 1988;**66**(6):1171-1180

[28] Guibourdenche J, Fournier T, Malassiné A, Evain-Brion D. Development and hormonal functions of the human placenta. Folia Histochemica et Cytobiologica. 2010;**47**(5):35-34

[29] Eriksson L, Frankenne F, Edèn S, Hennen G, Von Schoultz B. Growth hormone 24-h serum profiles during pregnancy—Lack of pulsatility for the secretion of the placental variant. Journal of Obstetrics and Gynaecology. 1989;**96**(8):949-953

[30] Hull KL, Harvey S. Growth hormone: Roles in female reproduction. Journal of Endocrinology. 2001;**168**(1):1-23

[31] Mazlan M et al. Circulating levels of-HGH-releasing hormone and HGH during human pregnancy. Journal of Endocrinology. 1990;**125**(1):161-167

[32] Lønberg U, Damm P, Andersson AM, Main KM, Chellakooty M, Lauenborg J, et al. Increase in maternal placental growth hormone during pregnancy and disappearance during parturition in normal and growth hormone-deficient pregnancies. American Journal of Obstetrics and Gynecology. 2003;**188**(1):247-251

[33] Randhawa R, Cohen P. The role of the insulin-like growth factor system in prenatal growth. Molecular Genetics and Metabolism. 2005;**86**(1-2):84-90

[34] Rosenfeld RG. Insulin-like growth factors and the basis of growth. The New England Journal of Medicine. 2003;**349**(23):2184-2186

[35] Curran AJ, Peacey SR, Shalet SM. Is maternal growth hormone essential for a normal pregnancy? European Journal of Endocrinology. 1998;**139**:54-58

[36] Giampietro A, Milardi D, Bianchi A, Fusco A, Cimino V, Valle D, et al. The effect of treatment with growth hormone on fertility outcome in eugonadal women with growth hormone deficiency: Report of four cases and review of the literature. Fertility and Sterility. 2009;**91**(3). DOI: 10.1016/j.fertnstert.2008.09.065

[37] Müller J, Starup J, Christiansen JS, Jøgensen JO, Juul A, Skakkebaek NE. Growth hormone treatment during pregnancy in a growth hormone-deficient woman. European Journal of Endocrinology. 1995;**132**(6):727-729. DOI: 10.1530/eje.0.1320727

[38] Wiren L, Boguszewski CL, Johannsson G. Growth hormone (GH) replacement therapy inHGH-deficient women during pregnancy. Clinical Endocrinology. 2002;**57**:235-239

[39] Vila G, Akerblad A, Mattsson AF, Riedl M, Webb SM. Pregnancy outcomes in women with growth hormone deficiency. Fertility and Sterility. 2015;**104**(5). DOI: 10.1016/j.fertnstert.2015.07.1132

[40] Alexander I, Anthony F, Letchworth AT. Placental protein profile and glucose studies in a normal pregnancy with extremely low levels of human placental lactogen: Case report. British Journal of Obstetrics and Gynaecology. 1982;**89**:241-243

[41] Barbieri F, Botticelli A, Consarino R, Genazzani AR, Volpe A. Failure of placenta to produce hPL in an otherwise uneventful pregnancy: A case report. Biological Research in Pregnancy and Perinatology. 1986;**7**:131-133

[42] Borody IB, Carlton MA. Isolated defect in human placental lactogen synthesis in a normal pregnancy. British Journal of Obstetrics and Gynaecology. 1981;**88**:447-449

[43] Bradford WP, Hargreaves T. Human placental lactogen in late pregnancy. Lancet. 1978;**3**:1213

[44] Gaede P, Trolle D, Pedersen H. Extremely low placental lactogen hormone (HPL) values in an otherwise uneventful pregnancy preceding delivery of a normal baby. Acta Obstetricia et Gynecologica Scandinavica. 1978;**57**:203-209

[45] Giampietro O, Ferdeghini M, Scatena P. Human placental lactogen (HPL) deficiency in a normal pregnancy. Postgraduate Medical Journal. 1984;**60**:689-690

[46] Hubert C, Descombey D, Mondon F, Daffos F. Plasma human chorionic somatomammotropin deficiency in a normal pregnancy is the consequence of low concentration of messenger RNA coding for human chorionic somatomammotropin. American Journal of Obstetrics and Gynecology. 1983;**147**:676-678

[47] Moshirpur J, Bernett A, McCarrick J, Allerhand J. hPL deficiency with normal estriol levels in a normal pregnancy. Obstetrics and Gynecology. 1981;**56**:65-85

[48] Nielsen PV, Pedersen H, Kampmann E-M. Absence of human placental lactogen in an otherwise uneventful pregnancy. American Journal of Obstetrics and Gynecology. 1979;**135**:322-326

[49] Parks JS, Nielsen PV, Sexton LA, Jorgensen EH. An effect of gene dosage on production of human chorionic somatomammotropin. The Journal of Clinical Endocrinology and Metabolism. 1985;**60**:994-997

[50] Sideri M, Virgiliis, de G, Giudobono F, Borgese N, Sereni LP, Nicolini U, et al. Immunologically undetectable human placental lactogen in a normal pregnancy: Case report. British Journal of Obstetrics and Gynaecology. 1983;**90**:771-773

[51] Simon P, Decoster C, Brocas H, Schwers J, Vassart G. Absence of human chorionic somatomammotropin during pregnancy associated with two types of gene deletion. Human Genetics. 1986;**74**:235-238

[52] Barrera-Saldaña HA. Origin of personalized medicine in pioneering, passionate, genomic research. Genomics. 10 May 2019. DOI: 10.1016/j.ygeno.2019.05.006. (In press)

[53] González-Rodríguez E, Jaramillo-Rangel G, Barrera-Saldaña HA. Molecular diagnosis of deletions in the human multi-gene complex of growth and placental lactogen hormones. American Journal of Medical Genetics. 1997;**72**(4):399-402

[54] Rygaard K, Revol A, Esquivel-Escobedo D, Beck BL, Barrera-Saldaña HA. Absence of human placental lactogen and placental growth hormone (HGH-V) during pregnancy: PCR analysis of the deletion. Human Genetics. 1998;**102**(1):87-92

[55] Wurzel JM, Parks JS, Herd JE, Nielsen PV. A gene deletion is responsible for absence of human chorionic somatomammotropin. DNA. 1982;**1**:251-257

[56] Ahangari GHASEM, Ostadali MR, Rabani A, Rashidian J, Sanati MH, Zarindast MR. Growth hormone antibodies formation in patients treated with recombinant human growth hormone. International Journal of Immunopathology and Pharmacology. 2004;**17**(1):33-38

[57] Johannsson G, Nespithal K, Plöckinger U, Alam V, McLean M. Multi-centre phase IV trial to investigate the immunogenicity of a new liquid formulation of recombinant human growth hormone in adults with growth hormone deficiency. Journal of Endocrinological Investigation. 2018;**41**(8):919-927

[58] Frisch H, Phillips JA 3rd. Growth hormone deficiency due to GH-N gene deletion in an Austrian family. Acta Endocrinologica. 1986;**279**:107-112

[59] Schwarz S, Berger P, Frisch H, Moncayo R, Phillips JA 3rd, Wick G. Growth hormone blocking antibodies in a patient with deletion of the GH-N gene. Clinical Endocrinology. 1987;**27**:213-224

[60] Hauffa BP, Illig R, Torresani T, Stolecke H, Phillips JA 3rd. Discordant immune and growth response to pituitary and biosynthetic growth hormone in siblings with isolated growth hormone deficiency type A. Acta Endocrinologica. 1989;**121**:609-614

[61] Riedl S, Frisch H. Effects of growth hormone (GH) and insulin-like growth factor-I therapy in patients with gene defects in the GH axis. Journal of Pediatric Endocrinology and Metabolism. 2006;**19**(3). DOI: 10.1515/jpem.2006.19.3.229

[62] Key NS. Inhibitors in congenital coagulation disorders. British Journal of Haematology. 2004;**127**:379-391

[63] Gilles JG, Desqueper B, Lenk H, Vermylen J, Saint-Remy JM. Neutralizing antiidiotypic antibodies to factor VIII inhibitors after desensitisation in patients with hemophilia A. The Journal of Clinical Investigation. 1996;**97**:1382-1388

[64] Van Parijs L, Abbas AK. Homeostasis and self-tolerance in the immune system: Turning lymphocytes off. Science. 1998;**280**:243-248

[65] Woods KA, Dastot F, Preece MA, Clark AJ, Postel-Vinay MC, Chatelain PG, et al. Phenotype: Genotype relationships in growth hormone insensitivity syndrome. The Journal of Clinical Endocrinology and Metabolism. 1997;**82**:3529-3535

[66] Burren CP, Woods KA, Rose SJ, Tauber M, Price DA, Heinrich U, et al. Clinical and endocrine characteristics in atypical and classical growth hormone insensitivity syndrome. Hormone Research. 2001;**55**:125-130

Chapter 6

Growth Hormone and Insulin-like Growth Factor-I: Novel Insights into the Male Reproductive Health

Mayank Choubey

Additional information is available at the end of the chapter

http://dx.doi.org/10.5772/intechopen.90710

Abstract

The roles of growth hormone (GH) in male reproductive health are summarized in this chapter. It has been evident in several studies that GH plays a vital physiological role in the regulation of male reproductive development and function, while the excessive release of GH can interfere with male reproductive health, sexual behavior, and fertility potentials. Several classical functions of GH include cellular proliferation, differentiation, development, and metabolism, although vast literature specifies their role in reproductive function in both humans and animals. Moreover, evidence from several studies have suggested both deficiency and overproduction of GH in adults are associated with several pathophysiological conditions, viz., metabolic derangements, central adiposity, dyslipidemia, and insulin resistance. The GH exerts its beneficial role by binding and activation to GH-receptors (GH-Rs), expressed at several target tissues, viz., in the hypothalamus and other parts of the central nervous system, and in the male gonad (testis), including Leydig and Sertoli cells. The GH may reflect either by local autocrine or paracrine actions or by the endocrine actions. The release of certain GH such as insulin-like growth factor 1 (IGF-1) plays a crucial role in the regulation of male reproductive physiology, while the excessive release of GH can interfere with male sexual behavior and fertility.

Keywords: growth hormone, IGF-1, male reproductive health, testicular metabolism, spermatogenesis, steroidogenesis

1. Introduction

Reproduction is the most essential process for any species to sustain its population. The reproductive health issues along with the infertility problems are observed very frequently nowadays. Approximately, 15% of all the couples trying to conceive are recognized as infertile,

IntechOpen

© 2020 The Author(s). Licensee IntechOpen. This chapter is distributed under the terms of the Creative Commons Attribution License (http://creativecommons.org/licenses/by/3.0), which permits unrestricted use, distribution, and reproduction in any medium, provided the original work is properly cited. cc BY

and the male partners are found to be solely responsible for half of all the cases of global childlessness [1]. In the recent time span, circa 20 years, the empirical developments have proved that several hypothalamic and pituitary hormones, including gonadotropin-releasing hormone (GnRH), growth hormone-releasing hormone (GH-RH), gonadotropins, and growth hormone (GH) and their corresponding canonic receptors, are ubiquitously and differentially expressed having diversity of biological functions [2]. There are myriad evidences showing that these vital endocrine hormones are also expressed in extra-hypothalamic and extra-pituitary tissues and are engaged in local synthesis and action, encompassing explicit effects on reproductive growth, cellular proliferation and survival, tissue repair, immunomodulation, cellular energy homeostasis and metabolism, antioxidative functions, and neuroregeneration [3–6]. It is manifested that GH synthesis is mainly through the pituitary somatotropes and is secreted as an endocrine hormone that regulates cellular growth and differentiation during testicular development [7]. Postnatally, GH pulsatile release is required as a homeostatic factor that in many tissues is indispensable for cellular proliferation and differentiation as well as the maintenance of their metabolic actions. The GH exerts its beneficial actions either by binding and activation to GH-receptors (GH-Rs), expressed at several target tissues, viz., in the hypothalamus and other parts of the central nervous system [8], and in the male gonad (testis), including Leydig and Sertoli cells [9]. As a pituitary endocrine hormone, growth hormone has cardinal roles in accentuating reproductive growth in individuals with GH deficiency [10]. Growth hormone deficiency (GHD) happens to be the most recurrent endocrinological abnormality, followed by gonadotropin, TSH, and ACTH deficiencies [11].

2. GH actions on the hypothalamic-pituitary-testicular (HPT) axis and male reproductive physiology

Gonadotropin-releasing hormone is considered to be the primary regulator of the male reproductive system, specifically controlling the pulsatile secretion of gonadotropins, i.e., luteinizing hormone (LH) and follicle-stimulating hormone (FSH) that are essential factors for proper gonadal activity [12]. Biosynthesis and release of GnRH are under complex excitatory and inhibitory control by a number of neurotransmitters and neurotrophic factors [13]. In addition, there are a number of autocrine/paracrine factors, including GH and insulin-like growth factor-1 (IGF-1), which can also modify the GnRH synthesis and action on the pituitary gonadotrophs, thereby influencing gonadal activity [10]. Here, we have attempted to summarize the influential evidence of GH/IGF-1 on male reproductive physiology and reproductive health. Although the central role of GH in growth and development is very well established in various tissues, GH's influence on male reproductive functions is poorly understood and requires thorough investigation.

2.1. Impact of GH on testicular growth, development, and pubertal maturation

Puberty is the multifaceted process through which children mature and develop secondary sexual characteristics and acquires reproductive competence. Normally pubertal transition is

http://dx.doi.org/10.5772/intechopen.90710

initiated through central mechanisms, with the gonadal function being driven by increased GnRH and gonadotropin secretion. Additionally, adequate energy supply and nutritional balance appear to be requisite for the central initiation of pubertal transition. At the testicular level, the GH promotes the growth and development of the gonad, in childhood and puberty, and stimulation of gametogenesis and production of steroid hormones, in puberty and reproductively mature period. The rate of GH synthesis doubles and attains a maximum peak during the pubertal maturation, and the production rate decreases with advancing age [14]. This mechanism is also supported by the IGF-1 produced in response to circulating GH levels. This is corroborated by studies that have shown the decrease in testicular volume in patients with childhood-onset growth hormone deficiency (CO-GHD) and the consequent increase in the same patients treated with replacement doses of GH [15]. GH also promotes the development and differentiation of internal testicular morphology such as seminiferous tubules (ST). In mammals, GH plays an imperative role to maintain normal sexual maturation, because puberty is deferred in GH-deficient [16, 17] or GH-resistant [15] humans. Analogously GH deficiency in rodents is associated with delayed sexual maturation [7, 18], and GnRH immunoneutralization delays sexual maturation in rats and reduces testicular mass, spermatogenesis, and follicle-stimulating hormone responsiveness [19]. The ability of GH to advance the pubertal maturation in GH-deficient children [20–23] and in GH-replete normal male rats [24] further illustrates the importance of GH in pubertal development. In some species, GH acts directly on androgen action, thereby accelerating the pubertal transition, because GH reduces the amount of testosterone required to induce secondary sexual characteristics (axillary hair) in young individuals [25].

2.2. Actions of GH on germ cell proliferation, survival, spermatogenesis, and sperm parameters

The impact of GH on testicular growth consequently influences the proliferation of germ cells. It is specifically an intricate point as it is a balance mechanism, whereby a decline in the levels of GH would lead to a simultaneous decrease in sperm count, semen volume, and sperm motility, respectively. It has been shown that surplus GH exerts the same consequences [24, 26, 27], highlighting the importance of the correct dosage of feasible therapies. Local IGF-1 may imitate GH effects on germ cells since sperm motility and morphology are recorded to be improved due to IGF-1 production. Receptors for IGF-1 are revealed in more mature haploid cells of spermatogenesis, i.e., secondary spermatocytes, spermatids, and spermatozoa as well. However, in some studies, the testicular level functions of these two entities have emphatically displayed antagonistic effects. Still, GH can act independently of IGF-1 [28]. These results illustrate the co-localization of GH and GH-RH in chicken testis and stimulatory function of GH-RH in testicular GH secretion along with a proliferation of testicular cells.

Beginning with the onset of puberty, spermatogenesis continues throughout the reproductively active periods in males. It is a highly complicated and conserved process, basically under the control of the HPG axis and intratesticular factors produced by Leydig and Sertoli cells. The hypothalamic decapeptide GnRH participates in the synthesis and release of gonadotropins, LH, and FSH into circulation by stimulating the anterior pituitary. Subsequently, these gonadotropins bind with their specific receptors, present/positioned on Leydig and Sertoli cells, leading to prompt production of steroids and other intratesticular factors required for spermatogenesis. With the aid of cell-to-cell signaling, these intratesticular factors regulate germ cell proliferation, survival, and apoptosis-inducing production of high-quality spermatozoa. A study conducted on the chicken elucidated the co-localization of GH and GH-RH in the testis and stimulatory roles of GH-RH in testicular GH secretion and in the proliferation of testicular cells. As a primal finding, testicular GH itself promotes testicular proliferation paving a definitive reason for proliferative action of GH-RH which is likely to be mediated through the autocrine/paracrine induction of GH secretion.

Improvement of sperm morphology and motility in GH-deficient dw/dw rats [29] and prolonged overall equine spermatozoa motility in vitro also hinges upon the GH, obtained possibly by extending sperm longevity [30]. Moreover, copious indicators of sperm quantity and quality in bulls are associated with GH gene polymorphisms [31]. Gametogenesis is similarly boosted up by GH in vitro cultures of eel testicular cells [28].

The spermatogenic actions of GH may be mediated by local IGF-I production since it can also revamp sperm motility and morphology [29], and GH coordinately augments IGF-I production in seminal vesicle and sperm motility [32]. However, few reports exhibit discordant effects of both GH and IGF-I [33], suggesting that GH may act exclusively of IGF-I. Similarly, the stimulatory effect of GH on eel spermatogenesis is not dependent on IGF-I and steroid [28].

The diminished, but not abolished, fertility in GH-resistant men and GH-deficient rodents [17, 19, 34] suggest that a low degree of fertility is felicitated by enough GH-independent local testicular IGF-I production. This phenomenon in chickens rather appears to be at an acceptable level to completely restore fertility parameters, since seminal IGF-I concentrations, sperm motility, morphology, viability, and fertility do not fluctuate between GH-resistant and GH-replete chickens [35].

2.3. Actions of GH in the modulation of testicular steroidogenesis

Steroidogenesis entails multistep processes that are enzyme-mediated and responsible for converting cholesterol into a biologically active steroid hormone. Regarding the hormonal feature of testicular function, GH is a potent steroidogenic factor, particularly in vitro. GH stimulates the production of androgen and/or estradiol by Leydig cells, isolated from rodents, ruminants, humans, and fish [7, 36], but not horses [37]. The results of in vivo studies are more contentious. While chronic GH therapy improves chorionic gonadotropin-induced testosterone production, some studies of fertile GH-deficient males [24, 38] and the testosterone response to hCG delineate attenuation in GH-R knockout mice [39]. Apparently, GH treatment in hypopituitary or moderately obese men actually decreases the concentrations of total serum testosterone [36, 37], potentially due to a stimulatory effect on aromatase activity and the resulting conversion of testosterone to estradiol observed in healthy young men treated with GH [40].

The reports from in vitro study demonstrate multifarious actions of GH, viz., alteration in the activity of enzymes involved in the steroidogenic pathway; stimulation of steroidogenic

http://dx.doi.org/10.5772/intechopen.90710

acute regulatory protein (StAR) production, which mediates cholesterol translocation across the inner mitochondrial membrane; and 3β-hydroxysteroid dehydrogenase (3β-HSD), which further converts pregnenolone into progesterone [18], in Leydig cell precursors of rodents. Similarly, GH upregulates the formation of early steroidogenic intermediates, such as 17-α 20-β dihydroprogesterone in testicular cells of fishes [41].

The gonadotrophic actions of GH may potentiate testicular steroidogenesis by promoting testicular LH sensitivity and enhancing Leydig cell proliferation and development, as GH-R knockout mice may be scarce in Leydig cells and LH receptors [39]. Similarly, GH is responsible for upregulation of LH receptors both in GH-replete (as in hamsters [42]) and GH-deficient (as in dwarf mice [43]) animals.

The bioavailability of free testosterone is curtailed because of the sex hormone-binding globulin (SHBG). Some studies corroborate that GH may potentiate testosterone activity by decreasing SHBG production. For instance, GH therapy minimizes SHBG levels in GH-deficient adults in some [37, 44], but not all [45] studies, and in hypopituitary adolescents [46]. Since the age-related decrease in SHBG concentration is not observed in GHD adolescents [47], therefore the pubertal rise in GH production may potentiate the male pubertal development.

However, ancillary studies in normal men reveal a coordinated decrease in sex hormone-binding globulin and total serum testosterone production following GH treatment [36], reduced SHBG but unaltered total serum testosterone [48], or increased LH-induced testosterone but unaltered SHBG [38]. These incongruities may reflect differences in subject age and GH administration protocol.

Some investigators have identified the importance of IGF-I in the steroidogenic actions of GH. IGF-I can imitate the effects of GH in rat testis [49] and partially reinstate testosterone synthesis in GH-resistant men [50]. Moreover, in another study conducted on rodents, GH-induced steroidogenesis required IGF-I co-administration [51]. However, de novo protein synthesis is redundant for GH-induced StAR synthesis, suggesting that at least a few testicular actions are IGF-I independent [18].

The earlier study observed a spontaneous correlation between testicular GH-R expression and StAR and p450 expression following exposure to nanoparticle-rich diesel exhaust (NR-DE) in rats [52]. However, much research work remains to be performed in order to identify a causal relationship between GH and pollutant-induced androgenesis.

2.4. Role of GH and IGF-I on the physiology of penile growth and erection

GH availability is imperative for penile growth since GH deficiency and GH resistance are frequently associated with micropenis and other penal anomalies [53]. Therefore, GH therapy improves penile growth in GH-deficient adolescents [54, 55]. IGF-I may mediate this very effect, since IGF-I administration to GH-resistant adolescents augments penile size, and this effect ceases when IGF-I therapy is withdrawn [50]. Similarly, in a study conducted on cultured postnatal foreskin fibroblasts cells, a stimulatory effect of IGF-I (but not GH) on the cellular proliferation of fibroblast was observed, independent to any changes in androgen receptors or 5-alpha reductase activity [55], whereas a more recent study, again conducted on fibroblast, noticed significant cellular growth and proliferation as a result of stimulatory effects of GH that was at least partially mediated by local IGF-I [56].

Contrarily, the erectile dysfunction may be due to altered autocrine/paracrine actions of GH, as erection requires relaxation of penile smooth muscle and modulation of blood flow. GH may facilitate both smooth muscle relaxation and systemic vasoconstriction. During penile tumescence in healthy men or men with psychogenic erectile dysfunction, the GH concentration in systemic and cavernous blood increases, but it is not so in the case of sexually aroused patients with organogenic erectile dysfunction [57–59]. An earlier study, conversely, did not observe any variations in systemic GH concentrations during sexual arousal and orgasm [60].

By stimulating the expression of neuronal nitric oxide synthase (nNOS) in intracavernosal nerves, GH is found to improve the erection frequency and maximal intracavernous pressure in aged rats [61, 62]. Next in order, GH also improves the regeneration of nNOS-expressing nerves following cavernous nerve neurotomy, accelerating the resumption of erectile function [63, 64]. This regenerative effect may involve local IGF-I and transforming growth factor beta-2 (TGF-β2), both of which were increased as a result of GH stimulation [65]. NOS may mediate important GH effects in humans, since GH, nitric oxide (NO), and cyclic guanosine monophosphate (cGMP) share a robust nexus in systemic and cavernous blood of individuals with erectile dysfunction [60]. GH also induces both relaxation and cGMP production in human cavernous strips [66]. However, a later study indicated that GH improves cGMP signaling in human corpora cavernosa (isolated from transsexual patients receiving hormonal therapy) independently of (NO) [67].

Since the pathophysiological GH concentrations in acromegalics are associated with erectile dysfunction, erectile effects of GH may be biphasic [68]. As libido is impaired in acromegalics [68] and boar's transgenic for the GH gene [69–72] as well as in GH-deficient males [73] and GH-R-knockout mice [74], the biphasic effects of GH on erectile function may partially reflect altered libido. Also, GH at optimum concentrations present in acromegalics stimulates contraction of dog corpus callosum strips [69].

2.5. Impact of GH/Insulin/IGF-1 signaling in the regulation of testicular metabolic and energy status

The GH stimulates the production of a family of proteins, viz., IGFs in several extrahepatic tissues including testis [75]. The IGFs composed predominantly of insulin, IGF1, IGF2, and their respective canonic receptors which upon activation provide signals to regulate a variety of cellular activities including cellular survival, proliferation, differentiation, and cellular metabolism [76, 77]. Importantly, testicular IGF-1 exerts its beneficial role by binding with its respective receptor and simultaneously activating it, in an autocrine/paracrine manner, and hence contributes to the maintenance of normal male reproductive physiology. Moreover, the earlier study utilizing IGF-1 null male mice showed infertile dwarf characteristics and also exhibit a reduction in both spermatogenic activity and serum levels of testosterone by ~80% [78]. This not only suggests the primary importance of GH/insulin/IGF signaling in body growth and development but also highlights its critical role in male reproductive health (**Figure 1**).

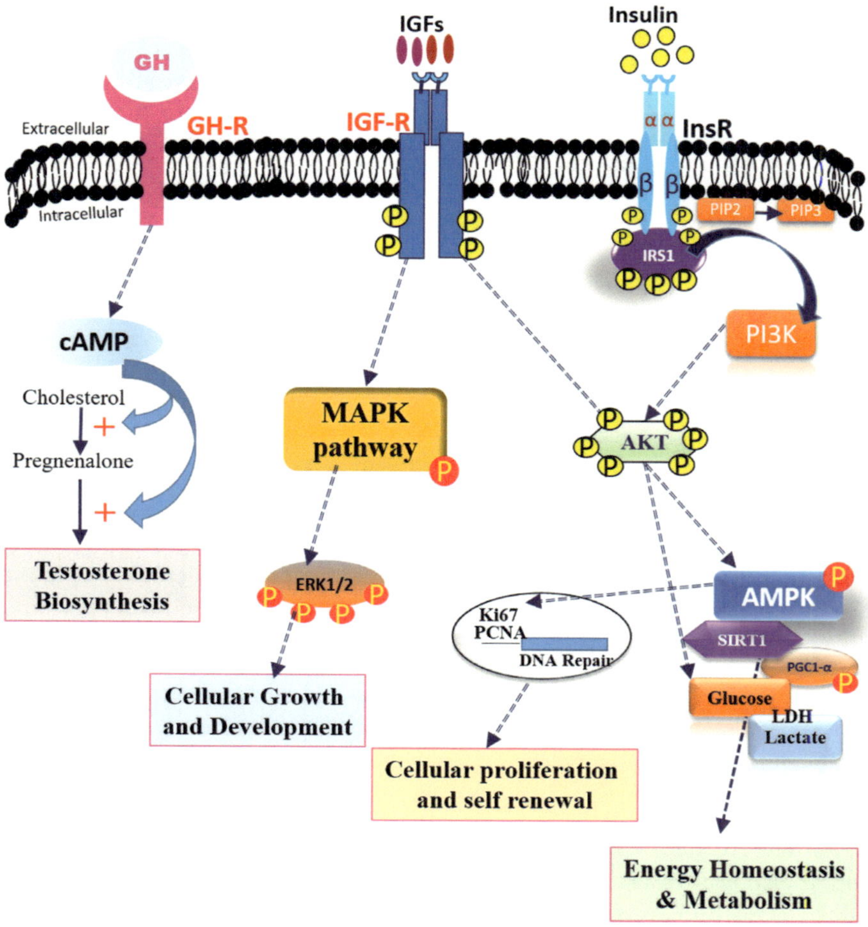

Figure 1. A schematic representation of GH/insulin/IGF signaling in the testicular axis. Both centrally (pituitary) and locally (testicular) secreted GH binds to the GH-receptors (GH-Rs) expressed in the Leydig cell and directly activates, releases secondary messenger i.e. cyclic adenosine monophosphate (cAMP), and stimulates (+) the activity of various steroidogenic enzymes (viz., StAR, p450scc, and 3β-HSD). Also it enhances the expression and abundance of luteinizing hormone receptor (LH-R) in the testis. The insulin/IGF1 signaling is mediated by a multifaceted, highly integrated network that regulates various crucial physiological processes. Two major signaling pathways are triggered by insulin/IGF1 activation, the ERK/MAPK pathway, and the ATK/PI3K/GLUT8 pathway, which are involved in numerous cellular processes such as cellular metabolism, cellular growth and proliferation, and self-renewal process of spermatogenic cells. Activation of the InsR/IGF-R signaling by insulin/IGF1/2 binding, respectively, leads to InsR (β subunits) as well as receptor tyrosine kinase phosphorylation, and this subsequently phosphorylates IRS proteins on their tyrosine residues, thereby activating the AKT/PI3K/GLUTs pathway. It is mainly responsible for the metabolic actions of insulin/IGF1 signaling (which activates the ERK/MAPK pathway and primarily regulates a variety of different downstream biological effects including mitogenesis, gene expression, and energy homeostasis by glucose and lactate transport to the developing germ cells).

Interestingly, GH-induced insulin/IGF family of growth factors activates glucose transporter 8 (GLUT8) which helps in chronological conversion of glucose into lactate by mature Sertoli cells [79, 80]. Notably, lactate is a preferred energy metabolite serving the energy requirement for proper testicular functioning and development of spermatogenic cells [81–83]. Also, the lactate production increases, as the Sertoli cell differentiates during pubertal development. It has been reported that the concentrations of lactate are low in the testes of the cryptorchid rat and intratesticular supplementation of lactate into the rats improves the development of haploid spermatozoa [84].

3. Therapeutic potentials of GH on reproductive health and male infertility

Male subfertility/infertility is a grave problem in the field of reproductive medicine. The growth hormone contributes to the restoration of sperm concentration, morphology, and motility in GH-deficient rats [85] and in men as well. The conventional remedy encompassing gonadotropin or pulsatile LH therapy may at times fail to generate the desired response. GH therapy proves to be a non-conventional adjuvant therapy which can be used to induce spermatogenesis in such non-responsive patients suffering with hypogonadotropic hypogonadism. A detailed study conducted on nine oligozoospermic and nine asthenozoospermic men treated with GH for 12 weeks reported increased sperm motility in both the groups, and three pregnancies were determined in asthenozoospermia, but not in oligozoospermia [86].

The administration of GH has been carried out as a possible treatment for infertility, due to the just mentioned potential to increase seminal volume and sperm motility [87], but there is still insufficient evidence that it can ameliorate sperm quality in patients with asthenozoospermia and oligozoospermia.

However, animal breeders and scientists focus mainly on the role of GH in milk and meat production; it also acts as a stimulant in anabolic processes. In modern research, the functions of the GH in human and animal reproduction have become an area of immense interest. As has already been empirically established, the process of gametogenesis in both sexes involves a vital role of GH, as it stimulates gamete production and maturation and embryo development as well. Although the GH activity modus operandi is still anonymous, GH therapy causes a considerable increase in sperm cell concentration, their motility, and IGF-1 content in the blood. The IGF-1 has proved to be the main GH mediator. Furthermore, tests have acknowledged an association between the rate of morphologically normal spermatozoa as well as IGF-1 concentration in seminal plasma. The discovery of active receptors in porcine testis and in bovine spermatozoa cells has ratified the action of GH and IGF-1 on sperm cells [88]. It is essentially required for determining the onset of puberty and the induction of sexual maturation. The regulation of growth and actions of secondary sexual organs and activation of the uterus in females and the seminal vesicles and prostate in males are its other spheres of activity. Its sphere of activity in adults consists of modulation of gonadotropin secretion and its exertion of gonadotropin-dependent and gonadotropin-independent actions on the local gonadal function, including steroidogenesis and gametogenesis.

4. Conclusion

GH is intimately involved in regulating reproductive physiology and maintenance of reproductive health in both the sexes. Although GH and IGFs are conventionally associated with growth and gonadotropin secretion, it has proven a pivotal role in several crucial processes associated with male reproductive health, i.e., sexual growth and differentiation, pubertal transition, spermatogenesis, gonadal steroidogenesis, metabolism, and sexual behavior. Besides being somatotropin, it is therefore considered as gonadotropin, integrally involved in male reproductive health. Despite plenteous reports showing the physiological functions of the somatotropic axis in male reproduction, the therapeutic implications are still very much obscure. The GH administration has been a pertinent approach in small groups of infertile males, but no controlled trial exists. However, the diagnosis of adult GHD is underestimated; it cannot solely be based on the measurement of circulating IGF-1 levels but requires exhaustive tests. In the case of reduced GH secretion, the replacement therapy can be proposed, especially in patients with oligozoospermia and low semen and testicular volume, which are passive towards gonadotropin administration. The role of GH as a modulator of testicular growth, differentiation, steroid synthesis, metabolism, and oxidative status is still a very interesting area to be explored. All these actions potentiate fertility status in both sexes and partially exhibit the neuroendocrine roles of pituitary GH, but as reproductive tissues are not just sites of GH action but also sites of local GH synthesis, they may reveal autocrine/paracrine actions of GH produced within the male reproductive system.

Author details

Mayank Choubey

Address all correspondence to: choubeymayank48@gmail.com

Department of Zoology, Institute of Science, Banaras Hindu University, Varanasi, Uttar Pradesh, India

References

[1] Inhorn MC, Patrizio P. Infertility around the globe: New thinking on gender, reproductive technologies and global movements in the 21st century. Human Reproduction Update. 2015;**21**:411-426. DOI: 10.1093/humupd/dmv016

[2] Martínez-Moreno CG, Calderón-Vallejo D, Harvey S, Arámburo C, Quintanar JL. Growth hormone (GH) and gonadotropin-releasing hormone (GnRH) in the central nervous system: A potential neurological combinatory therapy?. International Journal of Molecular Sciences. 2018;**19**:375. DOI: 10.3390/ijms19020375

[3] Cheung LW, Wong AS. Gonadotropin-releasing hormone: GnRH receptor signaling in extrapituitary tissues. The FEBS Journal. 2008;**275**:5479-5495

[4] Skinner DC, Albertson AJ, Navratil A, Smith A, Mignot M, Talbott H, et al. Effects of gonadotrophin-releasing hormone outside the hypothalamic-pituitary-reproductive axis. Journal of Neuroendocrinology. 2009;**21**:282-292

[5] Aguilar-Rojas A, Huerta-Reyes M. Human gonadotropin-releasing hormone receptor-activated cellular functions and signaling pathways in extra-pituitary tissues and cancer cells (review). Oncology Reports. 2009;**22**:981-990

[6] Harvey S. Extrapituitary growth hormone. Endocrine. 2010;**38**:335-359

[7] Sirotkin AV. Control of reproductive processes by growth hormone: Extra- and intracellular mechanisms. Veterinary Journal. 2005;**170**:307-317

[8] Nyberg F, Burman P. Growth hormone and its receptors in the central nervous system—Location and functional significance. Hormone Research. 1996;**45**:18-22

[9] Lobie PE, Breipohl W, Waters MJ. Growth hormone receptor expression in the rat gastrointestinal tract. Endocrinology. 1990;**126**:299-306

[10] Hull KL, Harvey S. Growth hormone and reproduction: A review of endocrine and autocrine/paracrine interactions. International Journal of Endocrinology. 2014;**2014**:234014. DOI: 10.1155/2014/234014

[11] Schoenmakers N, Alatzoglou KS, Chatterjee VK, Dattani MT. Recent advances in central congenital hypothyroidism. The Journal of Endocrinology. 2015;**227**(3):R51-R71. DOI: 10.1530/JOE-15-0341

[12] Marques P, Skorupskaite K, George JT, Anderson RA. Physiology of GNRH and gonadotropin secretion. In: Feingold KR, Anawalt B, Boyce A, et al., editors. Endotext. South Dartmouth (MA): MDText.com, Inc.; 2000

[13] Ciechanowska M, Lapot M, Mateusiak K, Przekop F. Neuroendocrine regulation of GnRH release and expression of GnRH and GnRH receptor genes in the hypothalamus-pituitary unit in different physiological states. Reproductive Biology. 2010;**10**:85-124

[14] Arsenijevic Y, Wehrenberg WB, Conz A, Eshkol A, Sizonenko PC, Aubert ML. Growth hormone (GH) deprivation induced by passive immunization against rat GH-releasing factor delays sexual maturation in the male rat. Endocrinology. 1989;**124**:3050-3059. DOI: 10.1210/endo-124-6-3050

[15] Rivarola MA, Heinrich JJ, Podestá EJ, De Chwojnik MF, Bergadá C. Testicular function in hypopituitarism. Pediatric Research. 1972;**6**:634-640

[16] Van-der-Werff-ten-Bosch JJ, Bot A. Growth of males with idiopathic hypopituitarism without growth hormone treatment. Clinical Endocrinology. 1990;**32**:707-717. DOI: 10.1111/j.1365-2265.1990.tb00917.x

[17] Stanhope R, Albanese A, Hindmarsh P, Brook CG. The effects of growth hormone therapy on spontaneous sexual development. Hormone Research. 1992;**1**:9-13. DOI: 10.1159/000182563

[18] Darendeliler F, Hindmarsh PC, Preece MA, Cox L, Brook CG. Growth hormone increases rate of pubertal maturation. Acta Endocrinologica (Copenhagen). 1990;**122**:414-416. DOI: 10.1530/acta.0.1220414

[19] Balducci R, Toscano V, Mangiantini A, Bianchi P, Guglielmi R, Boscherini B. The effect of growth hormone administration on testicular response during gonadotropin therapy in subjects with combined gonadotropin and growth hormone deficiencies. Acta Endocrinologica. 1993;**128**:19-23. DOI: 10.1530/acta.0.1280019

[20] Zachmann M, Prader A. Anabolic and androgenic affect of testosterone in sexually immature boys and its dependency on growth hormone. The Journal of Clinical Endocrinology and Metabolism. 1970;**30**:85-95. DOI: 10.1210/jcem-30-1-85

[21] Satoh K, Ohyama K, Nakagomi Y, Ohta M, Shimura Y, Sano T, et al. Effects of growth hormone on testicular dysfunction induced by cyclophosphamide (CP) in GH-deficient rats. Endocrine Journal. 2002;**49**(6):611-619. DOI: 10.1507/endocrj.49.611

[22] Nouri HS, Azarmi Y, Movahedin M. Effect of growth hormone on testicular dysfunction induced by methotrexate in rats. Andrologia. 2009;**41**(2):105-110. DOI: 10.1111/j.1439-0272.2008.00897.x

[23] Figueiredo MA, Fernandes RV, Studzinski AL, Rosa CE, Corcini CD, Junior AS, et al. GH overexpression decreases spermatic parameters and reproductive success in two-years-old transgenic zebrafish males. Animal Reproduction Science. 2013;**139**(1-4):162-167. DOI: 10.1016/j.anireprosci.2013.03.012

[24] Miura C, Shimizu Y, Uehara M, Ozaki Y, Young G, Miura T. Gh is produced by the testis of Japanese eel and stimulates proliferation of spermatogonia. Reproduction. 2011;**142**(6):869-877. DOI: 10.1530/REP-11-0203

[25] Vickers MH, Casey PJ, Champion ZJ, Gravance CG, Breier BH. IGF-I treatment increases motility and improves morphology of immature spermatozoa in the GH-deficient dwarf (dw/dw) rat. Growth Hormone & IGF Research. 1999;**9**:236-240. DOI: 10.1054/ghir.1999.0114

[26] Champion ZJ, Vickers MH, Gravance CG, Breier BH, Casey PJ. Growth hormone or insulin-like growth factor-I extends longevity of equine spermatozoa in vitro. Theriogenology. 2002;**57**(7):1793-1800. DOI: 10.1016/s0093-691x(02)00640-4

[27] Pal A, Chakravarty AK, Chatterjee PN. Polymorphism of growth hormone gene and its association with seminal and sexual behavioral traits in crossbred cattle. Theriogenology. 2014;**81**:474-480. DOI: 10.1016/j.theriogenology.2013.11.002

[28] Miao ZR, Lin TK, Bongso TA, Zhou X, Cohen P, Lee KO. Effect of insulin-like growth factors (IGFs) and IGF-binding proteins on in vitro sperm motility. Clinical Endocrinology. 1998;**49**:235-239. DOI: 10.1046/j.1365-2265.1998.00517.x

[29] Rowland JE, Kerr LM, White M, Noakes PG, Waters MJ. Heterozygote effects in mice with partial truncations in the growth hormone receptor cytoplasmic domain: Assessment of growth parameters and phenotype. Endocrinology. 2005;**146**:5278-5286. DOI: 10.1210/en.2005-0939

[30] Vergara M, Smith-Wheelock M, Harper JM, Sigler R, Miller RA. Hormone-treated snell dwarf mice regain fertility but remain long lived and disease resistant. The Journals of Gerontology. Series A, Biological Sciences and Medical Sciences. 2004;**59**:1244-1250. DOI: 10.1093/gerona/59.12.1244

[31] Zheng JX, Liu ZZ, Yang N. Deficiency of growth hormone receptor does not affect male reproduction in dwarf chickens. Poultry Science. 2007;**86**:112-117

[32] Singh MS, Joy KP. Effects of ovine LH, GH and prolactin, and testosterone on serum testosterone and estradiol-17β levels, and seminal vesicle and testicular activity in the catfish Clarias batrachus. Indian Journal of Experimental Biology. 2001;**39**:52-56

[33] Hess MF, Roser JF. A comparison of the effects of equine luteinizing hormone (eLH), equine growth hormone (eGH) and human recombinant insulin-like growth factor (hrIGF-I) on steroid production in cultured equine Leydig cells during sexual maturation. Animal Reproduction Science. 2005;**89**:7-19

[34] Carani C, Granata ARM, De-Rosa M, et al. The effect of chronic treatment with GH on gonadal function in men with isolated GH deficiency. European Journal of Endocrinology. 1999;**140**:224-230

[35] Deaver DR, Bryan KA. Effects of exogenous somatotropin (ST) on gonadal function in ruminants and swine. Domestic Animal Endocrinology. 1999;**17**:287-297

[36] Oscarsson J, Lindstedt G, Lundberg PA, Edén S. Continuous subcutaneous infusion of low dose growth hormone decreases serum sex-hormone binding globulin and testosterone concentrations in moderately obese middle-aged men. Clinical Endocrinology. 1996;**44**:23-29

[37] Giavoli C, Ferrante E, Ermetici F, et al. Effect of recombinant hGH (rhGH) replacement on gonadal function in male patients with organic adult-onset GH deficiency. Clinical Endocrinology. 2006;**65**:717-721

[38] Andreassen M, Frystyk J, Faber J, Kristensen LØ, Juul A. Growth hormone (GH) activity is associated with increased serum oestradiol and reduced anti-Müllerian hormone in healthy male volunteers treated with GH and a GH antagonist. Andrology. 2013;**1**:595-601

[39] Chandrashekar V, Bartke A, Awoniyi CA, Tsai-Morris CH, Dufau ML, Russell LD, et al. Testicular endocrine function in GH receptor gene disrupted mice. Endocrinology. 2001;**142**:3443-3450. DOI: 10.1210/endo.142.8.8298

[40] Kanzaki M, Morris PL. Growth hormone regulates steroidogenic acute regulatory protein expression and steroidogenesis in Leydig cell progenitors. Endocrinology. 1999;**140**:1681-1686. DOI: 10.1210/endo.140.4.6661

[41] Gac FL, Loir M. Control of testis function in fish: in vitro studies of gonadotropic regulation in the trout. Reproduction Nutrition Development. 1988;**28**:1031-1046

[42] Bex F, Bartke A, Goldman BD, Dalterio S. Prolactin, growth hormone, luteinizing hormone receptors, and seasonal changes in testicular activity in the golden hamster. Endocrinology. 1978;**103**:2069-2080

[43] Chatelain PG, Sanchez P, Saez GM. Growth hormone and insulin-like growth factor I treatment increase testicular luteinizing hormone receptors and steroidogenic responsiveness of growth hormone deficient dwarf mice. Endocrinology. 1991;**128**:1857-1862

[44] Gafny M, Silbergeld A, Klinger B, Wasserman M, Laron Z. Comparative effects of GH, IGF-I and insulin on serum sex hormone binding globulin. Clinical Endocrinology. 1994;**41**(2):169-175

[45] Juul A, Andersson AM, Pedersen SA, et al. Effects of growth hormone replacement therapy on IGF-related parameters and on the pituitary-gonadal axis in GH-deficient males. A double-blind, placebo-controlled crossover study. Hormone Research. 1998;**49**(6): 269-278

[46] Belgorosky A, Martinez A, Domene H, Heinrich JJ, Bergada C, Rivarola MA. High serum sex hormone binding globulin (SHBG) and low serum non-SHBG-bound testosterone in boys with idiopathic hypopituitarism: Effect of recombinant human growth hormone treatment. The Journal of Clinical Endocrinology and Metabolism. 1987;**65**:1107-1111

[47] Rudd BT, Rayner PH, Thomas PH. Observations on the role of GH/IGF-1 and sex hormone binding globulin (SHBG) in the pubertal development of growth hormone deficient (GHD) children. Acta Endocrinologica Supplementum. 1986;**279**:164-169

[48] Edén Engström B, Burman P, Johansson AG, Wide L, Karlsson FA. Effects of short-term administration of growth hormone in healthy young men, women, and women taking oral contraceptives. Journal of Internal Medicine. 2000;**247**:570-578

[49] Handelsman DJ, Spaliviero JA, Scott CD, Baxter RC. Identification of insulin-like growth factor-I and its receptors in the rat testis. Acta Endocrinologica. 1985;**109**:543-549

[50] Laron Z, Klinger B. Effect of insulin-like growth factor-I treatment on serum androgens and testicular and penile size in males with Laron syndrome (primary growth hormone resistance). European Journal of Endocrinology. 1998;**138**:176-180

[51] Laron Z, Sarel R. Penis and testicular size in patients with growth hormone insufficiency. Acta Endocrinologica. 1970;**63**:625-633

[52] Ramdhan DH, Ito Y, Yanagiba Y, Yamagishi N, Hayashi Y, Li C, et al. Nanoparticle-rich diesel exhaust may disrupt testosterone biosynthesis and metabolism via growth hormone. Toxicology Letter. 2009;**191**:103-108. DOI: 10.1016/j.toxlet.2009.08.013

[53] Laron Z, Mimouni F, Pertzelan A. Effect of human growth hormone therapy on penile and testicular size in boys with isolated growth hormone deficiency: First year of treatment. Israel Journal of Medical Sciences. 1983;**19**:338-344

[54] Levy JB, Husmann DA. Micropenis secondary to growth hormone deficiency: Does treatment with growth hormone alone result in adequate penile growth? The Journal of Urology. 1996;**156**:214-216

[55] Dykstra KD, Payne AM, Abdelrahim M, Francis GL. Insulin-like growth factor 1, but not growth hormone, has in vitro proliferative effects on neonatal foreskin fibroblasts without affecting 5-alpha-reductase or androgen receptor activity. Journal of Andrology. 1993;**14**(2):73-78

[56] Lee SW, Kim SH, Kim JY, Lee Y. The effect of growth hormone on fibroblast proliferation and keratinocyte migration. Journal of Plastic, Reconstructive & Aesthetic Surgery. 2010;**63**(4):e364-e369. DOI: 10.1016/j.bjps.2009.10.027

[57] Hamed EA, Meki AR, Gaafar AA, Hamed SA. Role of some vasoactive mediators in patients with erectile dysfunction: Their relationship with angiotensin-converting enzyme and growth hormone. International Journal of Impotence Research. 2003;**15**(6):418-425. DOI: 10.1038/sj.ijir.3901059

[58] Becker AJ, Uckert S, Stief CG, Scheller F, Knapp WH, Hartmann U, et al. Serum levels of human growth hormone during different penile conditions in the cavernous and systemic blood of healthy men and patients with erectile dysfunction. Urology. 2002;**59**(4):609-614

[59] Krüger T, Exton MS, Pawlak C, von zur Mühlen A, Hartmann U, Schedlowski M. Neuroendocrine and cardiovascular response to sexual arousal and orgasm in men. Psychoneuroendocrinology. 1998;**23**(4):401-411

[60] Zhang XS, Wang YX, Han YF, Li Z, Xiang ZQ, Leng J, et al. Effects of growth hormone supplementation on erectile function and expression of nNOS in aging rats. Zhonghua Nan Ke Xue. 2005;**11**(5):339-342

[61] Huang X, Hu LQ, Tian BQ. Growth hormone enhances regeneration of nNOS-containing nerve fibers in the aged rat penis. Zhonghua Nan Ke Xue. 2005;**11**(2):98-100

[62] Cui DS, Zhang KL, Pei F, Wei SZ, Hu LQ. Growth hormone enhances regeneration of cavernous nerves after their transplantation in rats. National Journal of Andrology. 2006;**12**:784-790

[63] Jung GW, Spencer EM, Lue TF. Growth hormone enhances regeneration of nitric oxide synthase-containing penile nerves after cavernous nerve neurotomy in rats. Journal of Urology. 1998;**160**(5):1899-1904

[64] Jung GW, Kwak JY, Yoon S, Yoon JH, Lue TF. IGF-I and TGF-beta2 have a key role on regeneration of nitric oxide synthase (NOS)-containing nerves after cavernous neurotomy in rats. International Journal of Impotence Research. 1999;**11**(5):247-259

[65] Becker AJ, Uckert S, Stief CG, Truss MC, Machtens S, Scheller F, et al. Possible role of human growth hormone in penile erection. The Journal of Urology. 2000;**164**(6): 2138-2142

[66] Uckert S, Scheller F, Stief CG, Knapp WH, Sohn M, Becker AJ, et al. Potential mechanism of action of human growth hormone on isolated human penile erectile tissue. Urology. 2010;**75**(4):968-973. DOI: 10.1016/j.urology.2009.05.046.

[67] Jadresic A, Banks LM, Child DF, Diamant L, Doyle FH, Fraser TR, et al. The acromegaly syndrome. Relation between clinical features, growth hormone values and radiological characteristics of the pituitary tumours. The Quarterly Journal of Medicine. 1982;**51**(202):189-204

[68] Ra S, Aoki H, Fujioka T, Sato F, Kubo T, Yasuda N. In vitro contraction of the canine corpus cavernosum penis by direct perfusion with prolactin or growth hormone. The Journal of Urology. 1996;**156**:522-525

[69] Rejduch B, Słota E, Sysa P, Rózycki M. Reproductive performance of a transgenic boar carrying the bovine growth hormone gene (bGH). Journal of Applied Genetics. 2002;**43**(3):337-341

[70] Pursel VG, Bolt DJ, Miller KF, Pinkert CA, Hammer RE, Palmiter RD, et al. Expression and performance in transgenic pigs. Journal of Reproduction and Fertility. Supplement. 1990;**40**:235-245

[71] Pinkert CA, Kooyman DL, Dyer TJ. Enhanced growth performance in transgenic swine. Biotechnology. 1991;**16**:251-258

[72] Fujita K, Terada H, Ling LZ. Male sexual insufficiency. Nippon Rinsho. 1997;**55**:2908-2913

[73] Bartke A. Role of growth hormone and prolactin in the control of reproduction: What are we learning from transgenic and knock-out animals? Steroids. 1999;**64**:598-604

[74] Liu JL, Yakar S, LeRoith D. Conditional knockout of mouse insulin-like growth factor-1 gene using the Cre/loxP system. Proceedings of the Society for Experimental Biology and Medicine. 2000;**223**(4):344-351

[75] Griffeth RJ, Bianda V, Nef S. The emerging role of insulin-like growth factors in testis development and function. Basic and Clinical Andrology. 2014;**24**:1-10. DOI: 10.1186/2051-4190-24-12

[76] Efstratiadis A. Genetics of mouse growth. The International Journal of Developmental Biology. 1998;**42**:955-976

[77] Nakae J, Kido Y, Accili D. Distinct and overlapping functions of insulin and IGF-I receptors. Endocrine Reviews. 2001;**22**:818-835

[78] Baker J, Hardy MP, Zhou J, Bondy C, Lupu F, Bellve AR, et al. Effects of an Igf1 gene null mutation on mouse reproduction. Molecular Endocrinology. 1996;**10**:903-918

[79] Escott GM, de Castro AL, Jacobus AP, Loss ES. Insulin and IGF-I actions on IGF-I receptor in seminiferous tubules from immature rats. Biochimica et Biophysica Acta. 2014;**1838**(5):1332-1337. DOI: 10.1016/j.bbamem.2014.02.002

[80] Rato L, Alves MG, Socorro S, Duarte AI, Cavaco JE, Oliveira PF. Metabolic regulation is important for spermatogenesis. Nature Reviews. Urology. 2012;**9**(6):330-338. DOI: 10.1038/nrurol.2012.77

[81] Choubey M, Ranjan A, Bora PS, Baltazar F, Krishna A. Direct actions of adiponectin on changes in reproductive, metabolic, and anti-oxidative enzymes status in the testis of adult mice. General and Comparative Endocrinology. 2019;**279**:1-11. DOI: 10.1016/j.ygcen.2018.06.002

[82] Choubey M, Ranjan A, Bora PS, Baltazar F, Martin LJ, Krishna A. Role of adiponectin as a modulator of testicular function during aging in mice. Biochimica et Biophysica Acta—Molecular Basis of Disease. 2019;**1865**(2):413-427. DOI: 10.1016/j.bbadis.2018.11.019

[83] Choubey M, Ranjan A, Bora PS, Krishna A. Protective role of adiponectin against testicular impairment in high-fat diet/streptozotocin-induced type 2 diabetic mice. Biochimie. 2019;**168**:41-52. DOI: 10.1016/j.biochi.2019.10.014

[84] Courtens JL, Plöen L. Improvement of spermatogenesis in adult cryptorchid rat testis by intratesticular infusion of lactate. Biology of Reproduction. 1999;**61**(1):154-161

[85] Gravance CG, Breier BH, Vickers MH, Casey PJ. Impaired sperm characteristics in postpubertal growth-hormone-deficient dwarf (dw/dw) rats. Animal Reproduction Science. 1997;**49**:71-76

[86] Ovesen P, Jørgensen JO, Ingerslev J, Ho KK, Orskov H, Christiansen JS. Growth hormone treatment of subfertile males. Fertility and Sterility. 1996;**66**:292-298

[87] Ovesen PG, Jørgensen JO, Ingerslev J, Orskov H, Christiansen JS. Growth hormone treatment of men with reduced sperm quality. Ugeskrift for Laeger. 1998;**160**:176-180

[88] Machnik G, Lechniak D. The impact of growth hormone (GH) on male reproduction. Medycyna Weterynaryjna. 2000;**56**:218-221

Section 3

Acromegaly

Chapter 7

Pegvisomant in Acromegaly and Gigantism

Claire Briet, Valentine Suteau and Patrice Rodien

Additional information is available at the end of the chapter

http://dx.doi.org/10.5772/intechopen.91251

Abstract

Pegvisomant is a GH antagonist used in acromegaly in gigantism. Pegvisomant is a modified GH molecule with pegylation to increase half-life and nine amino acid substitutions to modify GH receptor affinity and dimerization. Pegvisomant leads to an IGF1 decrease. It is administered subcutaneously every day with a median dose of 15 mg/day in meta-analysis. This treatment is indicated in acromegaly or gigantism in case of resistance to somatostatin analogs. This drug leads to a control of acromegaly in 90% of patients in phase III study and about 70% of patients in real-life study. In gigantism, only 50% of children are controlled with pegvisomant. It is a well-tolerated treatment with hepatic side effects in 3% of cases, headache in 2% of cases, and lipohypertrophy in 3% of cases. Pegvisomant does not act on adenoma size, and 6% of increasing tumour size is observed. Indeed, pegvisomant is an antagonist of GH receptor with a good efficacy which can be used alone or in association with somatostatin analog or cabergoline if acromegaly is not controlled by a somatostatin analog.

Keywords: acromegaly, gigantism, pegvisomant

1. Introduction

Pegvisomant is the only available GH antagonist. The history of pegvisomant development is an example of how research can be surprising. By combining site-specific mutation on the GH gene, researchers were looking for a long-acting GH treatment. However, researchers were surprised to find with the in vivo analysis an IGF1 reduction in mice treated with the modified GH molecule obtained. It was the beginning of pegvisomant history.

IntechOpen

© 2020 The Author(s). Licensee IntechOpen. This chapter is distributed under the terms of the Creative Commons Attribution License (http://creativecommons.org/licenses/by/3.0), which permits unrestricted use, distribution, and reproduction in any medium, provided the original work is properly cited. (cc) BY

2. Structure-function

2.1. Development of a long-acting GH antagonist

GH three-dimensional structure contains two disulphide bridges and four helices which are arranged in an "up-up-down-down" topology. Helices 1, 2, 3, and 4 are located between residues 9–34, 72–92, 106–128, and 155–184, respectively (**Figure 1**) [1]. Helix 3 is the key to promote a growth activity. In this helix, approximately 20 amino acids are arranged in an amphiphilic orientation. Among them, three amino acids do not enable an ideal amphiphilic helix [2]. When modifying these three amino acids, researchers wanted to generate a perfect amphiphilic helix 3 and hypothesised that it would enhance GH activity. Surprisingly, transgenic mice expressing this modified GH analog had decreased circulating IGF1 concentrations. It was the first report of a GH antagonist [3]. Further single amino acid substitutions demonstrated that glycine at position 120 of human GH was critical for the growth-promoting activity of the respective molecule. Crystallography studies demonstrated that this mutation of the glycine to a lysine at position 120 (G120K) of GH led to a defect of GHR dimerisation which is essential for GH transduction signal [4].

However, because of its small size (22 kDa), GH is rapidly cleared by the kidneys and/or endocytosis as a GH/GHR complex. Indeed, the addition of polyethylene glycol (PEG) (5 kDa)

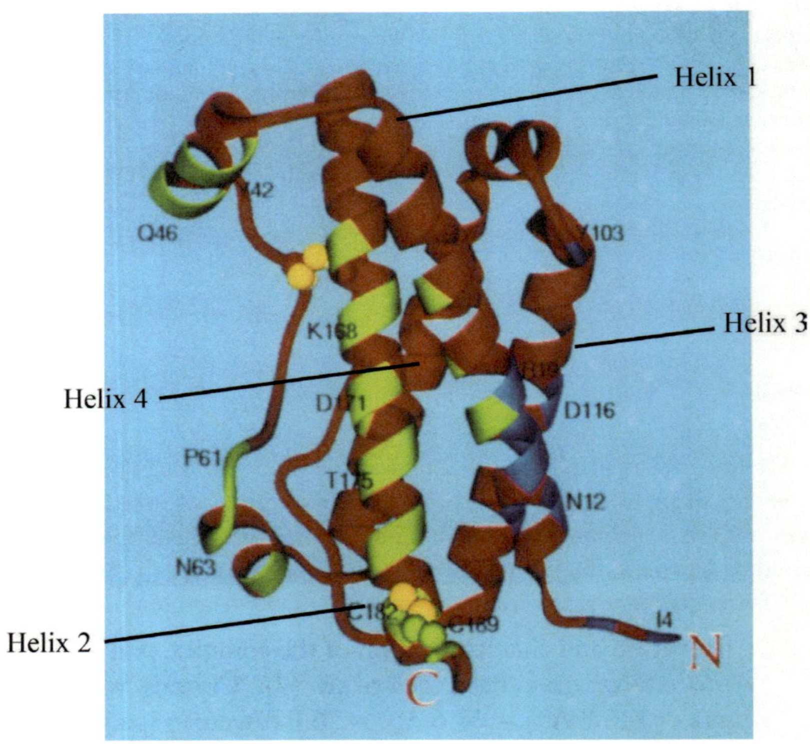

Figure 1. Two-dimensional representation of the structure of human GH (adapted from de Vos et al.) [4].

increased the serum half-life from 30 min to 2 days. At this stage, we had a G120K-PEG GH molecule. However, the perfect GH antagonist was not yet found because the addition of PEG led to a decrease of binding affinity for site 1 (which is the first binding site of the GH molecule on the GH receptor). To circumvent this problem, mutagenesis of binding site 1 was considered. In the meantime, Cunningham and Wells published a more potent GH analog with eight amino acid substitutions in site 1 of the GH molecule. These eight mutations were introduced in the G120K-PEG GH molecule [5]. This molecule proved to maintain binding affinity for binding site 1 of GHR, antagonising properties of GHR with a long half-life. That was the birth of pegvisomant.

2.2. The pegvisomant/GHR interaction

Pegvisomant/GHR interaction has been more precisely studied. Primary studies suggest that pegvisomant binds to one GHR and prevents GHR dimerisation because of the G120K mutation which prevents binding to site 2. However, further studies show that pegvisomant

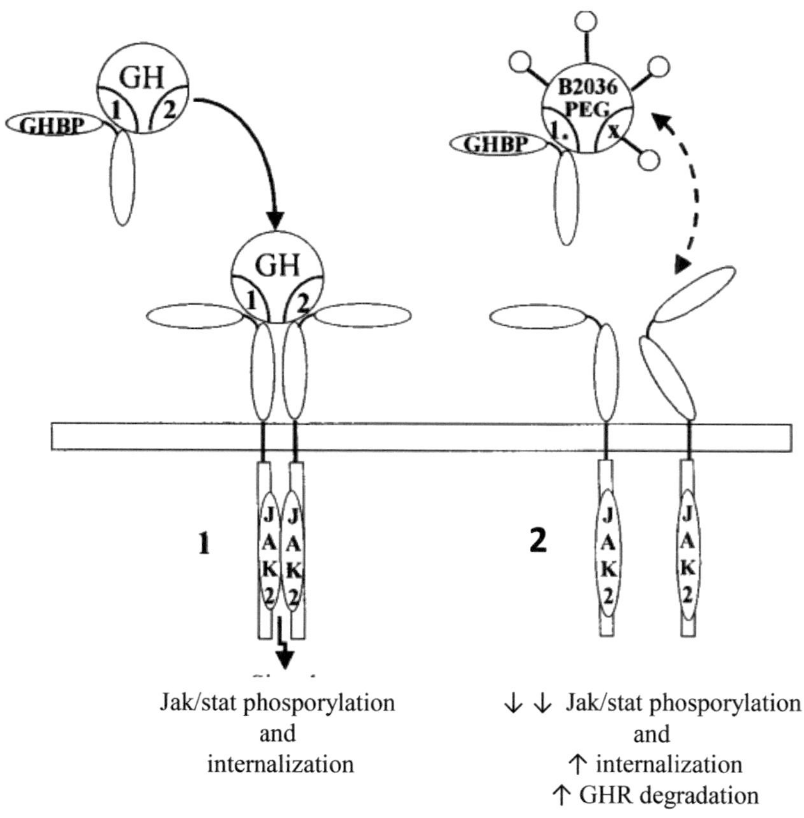

Figure 2. Binding representation of GH and pegvisomant (B2036-PEG) on GH receptor and schematic effect [1]. GH binds to GHBP and to binding site 1 and 2, inducing a conformational change of GHR, a jak/stat phosphorylation, and internalisation [2]. Pegvisomant binds to GHBP, and the complex binds to site 1 and site 2, inducing a less functional dimerization, a diminution of jak/stat phosphorylation, and a different intracellular trafficking with an increase of GH receptor degradation (adapted from Ross et al.) [6].

induces GHR dimerisation with disulphide linkage and induces internalisation, as GH do. However, activation of jak kinase and stat 5 is less important because the conformation changes after pegvisomant binding is different with a less functional dimerisation [6, 7]. Moreover, internalisation after pegvisomant binding induces a different intracellular trafficking, with an increase of degradation of GHR, a decrease of GHR expression on cellular membrane, and a decrease of nuclear localisation of GHR [8].

Moreover, it appears that the eight mutations within site 1 do not increase affinity to GHR but to the GH binding protein and allow the dimerisation of GHR despite the pegylation (**Figure 2**) [7]. Reducing site 1 binding affinity, high doses of pegvisomant are necessary to antagonise GH action.

3. Safety-efficacy

3.1. Phase I

In the phase I study, 36 young volunteers received a single injection of either the placebo or pegvisomant (0.03, 0.1, 0.3, or 1.0 mg/kg). All doses were well tolerated, with no severe adverse events. IGF1 decreased significantly in all groups with a pegvisomant dose above 0.1 mg/kg ($P < 0.001$ vs. placebo) [9].

3.2. Phase II

In the phase II study, 46 patients with active acromegaly were randomised and received the placebo, 30 or 80 mg of pegvisomant once a week for 6 weeks. If IGF1 levels were unchanged in the placebo group, it decreased by 31 ± 6.7% in the 80 mg groups ($P < 0.001$). There was a dose-related decrease in serum IGF1. However, only three patients have a normal serum IGF1. Pharmacokinetic study evaluated pegvisomant half-life at 70 h [10]. Because of the low efficacy of pegvisomant in phase II and the half-life of 70 h, it was decided to give pegvisomant daily in phase III.

3.3. Phase III

The phase III study on 112 patients with acromegaly showed the efficacy of pegvisomant on serum IGF1 reduction and clinical improvement. This double-blind study showed a decrease of IGF1 from the baseline by 26.7 ± 27.9%, 50.1 ± 26.7%, and 62.5 ± 21.3% in the groups that received 10 mg, 15 mg, and 20 mg of pegvisomant per day, respectively ($P < 0.001$ for the comparison of each pegvisomant group with placebo). In these groups, 54%, 81%, and 89% had a normalised IGF1 at 12 weeks. Among patients treated with 15 mg or 20 mg of pegvisomant per day, there were significant decreases in clinical symptoms such as ring size, soft tissue swelling, the degree of excessive perspiration, and fatigue. Quality of life improved in all groups. Tumour volume was similar before pegvisomant and at 12 weeks [11]. One year later, van der Lely et al. published the extension of this study, with 152 patients on pegvisomant at 18 months; 97% of patient normalised serum IGF1 (**Table 1**) [12].

http://dx.doi.org/10.5772/intechopen.91251

	N (female)	IGF1 before pegvisomant % ULN	Median exposure time (months)	Median dose mg/day (min max)	Monotherapy (% of patients)	Normal IGF1 (% of patients)	Tumour enlargement (% of patients)	Liver enzyme elevation (% of patients)
Boguszewski et al. [14]	109 (61)	209 (99–637)	30.5	10 (10–30)	11	74.1%	6	9.2
Basavilbaso et al. [33]	75 (51)	240 (125–700)	27	12 (3–30)	45	63%	9.8	9.3
Buchfelder et al. [13]	2090	NA	91.2	18.9	NA	73	2.2	3
Van der Lely et al. [12]	90	NA	18	19.6	100	97	1.3	1.3
Garcia et al. [18]	42	NA	NA	NA	NA	58	NA	NA
Rostomyan et al. [19]	37	NA	NA	NA	NA	51	NA	NA

NA: not available; ULN: Upper limit normal.

Table 1. Main study of pegvisomant efficacy and adverse events in real life.

3.4. Long-term experience

3.4.1. *Efficacy*

The ACROSTUDY is the largest international, noninterventional study of acromegaly patients treated by pegvisomant. Two thousand and ninety patients were analysed between 2004 and 2016. When starting pegvisomant, 89% of patients had an IGF1 above the upper limit of normal (ULN), previously treated by surgery, radiotherapy, medical therapy, or a combination of the three. After 10 years, 73% of patients had a normal IGF1 with a median dose of pegvisomant 18.9 mg/day (**Table 1**) [13].

A recent study evaluated the efficacy in real life. A Brazilian multicentre study of 109 patients with acromegaly were included, 61% were women, and 95% have macroadenomas. Previous treatments were surgery (89%), radiotherapy (34%), somatostatin analogs (99%), and/or cabergoline (67%). No patients were controlled at inclusion with high IGF1 (median 209% of ULN) and high GH secretion. For most patients the initial dose was 10 mg/day, and the median exposure was 30.5 months. Pegvisomant was used as monotherapy in 11%. IGF1 normalisation was obtained in 74% of patients with a median dose of 15 mg/day when used alone and 10 mg/day in combined therapy. In this study, there were three response predictors: exposure time, GH pretreatment, and IGF1 pretreatment (**Table 1**) [14].

In a recent meta-analysis of eight studies, 60.9% of patients were controlled (52–70; 95% CI) and 72% if considering only patients in monotherapy in five studies [15].

Interestingly, there are two cases of persistent remission of acromegaly after pegvisomant withdrawal. Patients were treated for 8 and 11 years and presented a normal IGF1 and GH secretion 5 and 2 years after withdrawal, respectively [16].

3.4.2. Adherence

In a recent study, treatment adherence to pegvisomant was evaluated in a multicentre cross-sectional study on patients treated with pegvisomant for more than 12 months in 108 patients. Rates of adherence varied from 61 to 92% and did not correlate to disease control. Older patients and patients with an alternative schedule had lower adherence. However, treatment satisfaction was high, 75 ± 15%, evaluated with the "Treatment Satisfaction with Medicines Questionnaire" (STATMED-Q). This study reveals that the principal obstacle was the transportation of the pegvisomant (especially maintaining the cold chain during transportation) and anxiety about the injection. One third of patients made mistakes during the reconstitution (17%) and administration (22%) of pegvisomant [17].

3.5. Experience of pegvisomant in children

Experience of pegvisomant in children is quite rare. There is a recent review of the case series of gigantism in the literature. Out of 262 patients, 42 (17.5%) were treated with pegvisomant and 27 (58%) had normal IGF1 [18]. The biggest series was published in 2015 with 208 patients with gigantism. Among them 37 were treated with pegvisomant and 19/37 (51%) had a normal IGF1. Indeed, gigantism seems to be more difficult to control than acromegaly in adulthood with pegvisomant [19].

4. Indication

4.1. Acromegaly patients

Endocrine society guidelines for acromegaly were published in 2014 [20]. The first recommended treatment of acromegaly is surgery, as it offers the prospect of a cure. In case of persistent GH secretion 12 weeks after surgery, medical treatment is indicated including cabergoline and long-acting somatostatin (SMS) analogs. Cabergoline is indicated in case of co-secretion of GH and PRL or if GH secretion is slightly increased (IGF1 < 2.5 times the upper normal range) and permits 40–50% of control [21, 22]. The first generation of long-acting SMS analog studies report around 50% of IGF1 normalisation [23]. For patients who are not controlled by the first-generation SMS analogs, the recent consensus recommends several options:

Add cabergoline if IGF1 is <2.5 times the upper normal range.

Switch to pasireotide, the second-generation of SMS analogs which normalised IGF1 in up to 54% of patients [24].

Switch or add pegvisomant [25].

Pegvisomant is indicated in cases of resistance to SMS analog in a second- or third-line therapy [20]. In addition, pegvisomant should be considered in patient with uncontrolled diabetes with partial or no response to first-line medical therapy [25].

4.2. Posology

For the first dose, 80 mg is recommended, followed by 10 mg/day. IGF1 should be measured 8 weeks after, and pegvisomant should be increased by stages of 5 mg.

The dose of pegvisomant required to normalise IGF1 can be evaluated with age and BMI; however, it is recommended to monitor IGF1 in order to adapt pegvisomant dosage. Using dose above 30 mg/day is not recommended [26].

4.3. Combination therapy

When patients are not controlled with somatostatin analog ± cabergoline, the question of adding pegvisomant or switching to pegvisomant is not yet resolved. Initially, with serum IGF1 normalisation in over 90% of patients with acromegaly receiving pegvisomant, the indications for combined therapy were limited. However, in real life, as efficacy is lower (almost 70%), the combination therapy is questionable. Moreover, because of the risk of tumour growth and chiasma compression, the strategy for macroadenoma was often to add pegvisomant to somatostatin analog. However, the routine use of SMS analog and pegvisomant in combination may also be prohibitively expensive [27].

A randomised trial compared the two strategies for patients uncontrolled under long-acting octreotide: switched to pegvisomant alone or added pegvisomant. IGF1 normalisation was similar in both groups (56% for pegvisomant alone and 62% for combined therapy). The question still remains unanswered [28].

In a large Dutch cohort of patients with acromegaly treated with the association of somatostatin analog and pegvisomant for 9 years, 97% of patients had a normal IGF1 with a median dose of pegvisomant of 80 mg/week [29].

Moreover, the association of cabergoline and pegvisomant for patients with a slightly increase of IGF1 under pegvisomant alone for 18 months enabled acromegaly control in four patients (28%) [22].

4.4. Monitoring and objectives

IGF1 is the only biological marker to evaluate disease activity on pegvisomant. As it is a GH antagonist, it is not recommended to follow GH secretion. Indeed, scoring systems have been developed to evaluate the activity of acromegaly. In this way, SAGIT and ACRODAT are additional tools to assess overall disease activity [30, 31]. AcroQol can be useful to evaluate the quality of life of acromegaly patient under treatment [32].

5. Adverse events

5.1. Hepatic

In the phase III study, one patient with 15 mg/day of pegvisomant withdrew after 8 weeks of therapy because of elevated serum aminotransferase levels, with a normalisation of liver function after withdrawal. In this patient, serum alanine aminotransferase and aspartate aminotransferase rose to 20 N and 10 N, respectively. In the cohort of patients receiving pegvisomant, mean serum aminotransferase levels were stable (n = 80) [11].

In the Brazilian and Argentinian cohort, elevation of liver enzymes was reported in 9% of cases and was responsible for pegvisomant discontinuation in 1 and 5 patients, respectively (**Table 1**) [14, 33].

A recent meta-analysis of 6 studies with pegvisomant in monotherapy showed an overall rate of transaminase elevation of 3.0% (1.7–5.2%; 95% CI; I 2 = 55%) (**Table 1**) [15].

5.2. Headache

In the phase III study, one patient with 15 mg/day of pegvisomant withdrew due to persistent headaches [11]. In the Brazilian real-life study, headaches were reported in two cases (1.8%) [14].

5.3. Cutaneous lipohypertrophy

In the phase III study, injection site reactions were reported in six patients (5%) receiving pegvisomant [11]. In the Brazilian real-life study, it was reported in 4.6% of patients [14]. Pain from injection was reported in 2.7% patients.

In the Argentinian cohort, 3 out of 75 patients had localised lipodystrophy [33].

A recent meta-analysis of five studies with pegvisomant showed lipohypertrophy in 1.6% of patients (0.6–4.3%; 95% CI; I 2 = 69%) [15].

5.4. Antibody formation

Because of the nine amino acid substitutions, pegvisomant is different from GH and can be considered as foreign protein leading to an immunoreactivity. Pegylation of the molecule reduces immunogenicity. However, in the phase III study and its extension, anti-GH antibodies were reported in 8/112 (7%) patients between 1:14 and 1:64 and pegvisomant antibody in 16.9% [12, 15].

5.5. Metabolic

Several studies evaluated glucose metabolism in patients with pegvisomant. In 53 patients initially treated by long-acting octreotide, the switch for pegvisomant treatment induced normalisation of IGF1 in 78% of cases at 32 weeks and a significant diminution of median fasting glucose (1.4 mmol/l) and HbA1C (−0.2%) whatever the diabetes and IGF1 status. In the subgroup of diabetic patients, a significant decrease of HbA1C (−1%) was observed [34].

In the ACROSTUDY, among the 1762 patients, 29% had diabetes before pegvisomant. At year 4, mean fasting blood glucose decreased from 140 ± 59 to 120 ± 44 mg/dl, and the decrease of HbA1C was not significant whatever the diabetes status [35].

In a recent meta-analysis, pegvisomant significantly decreased fasting blood glucose level (−0.8 mmol/l; 95% CI; −1.0 to −0.6), fasting insulin level (−5.31; 95% CI; −10.2 to −0.4), and

HbA1c (−0.43%; 95% CI; −0.6 to −0.3). Indeed, HOMA-I also decreased −0.61 (95% CI; −1.2 to −0.04). This increase in glucose metabolism was not correlated to IGF1 level [36].

5.6. Tumour size

In the ACROSTUDY, subjects received pegvisomant for a mean of 5.4 years, and 12 out of 542 subjects (2.2%) had a confirmed increase in tumour size (**Table 1**) [37].

In the Brazilian study, tumour enlargement was reported in 6.5% of cases (n = 5). In the Argentinian study, 4 of 50 patients (8%) showed an increase in tumour size with pegvisomant (**Table 1**) [33]. In the meta-analysis of five studies with pegvisomant in monotherapy, the overall tumour growth rate was 7.2% (4.8–10.7%; 95% CI; I 2 = 0%) [15].

5.7. Bones

The bone is a well-known fragility key point in acromegaly with a high incidence of vertebral fractures [38]. A recent study evaluated vertebral fracture in 55 patients resistant to the first generation of somatostatin analogs. Before introducing pasireotide or pegvisomant, vertebral fracture occurred in 23 patients (42%). In uncontrolled acromegaly, there were 78% of vertebral fractures under pegvisomant and 25% under pasireotide (p = 0.04). In controlled acromegaly, there were 23% of vertebral fractures under pegvisomant and 12.5% under pasireotide (p = 0.4). Indeed, vertebral fractures seem to be more frequent with pegvisomant [39].

However, another longitudinal study has a different result in 83 patients treated with somatostatin analog alone (42 cases), pegvisomant alone (6 cases), or in combination with somatostatin analog (35 cases) for a median period of 82 months (range 36–126). In this longitudinal study, the authors observed a global decrease in incidence of radiological vertebral fractures from 43.9 to 26.8% (p = 0.039). For patients treated by pegvisomant, the incidence of vertebral fractures was not significantly decreased as compared to patients treated with somatostatin analog (10.0 vs. 26.7%; p = 0.09). In this study, pegvisomant did not increase vertebral fractures [40].

6. Conclusion

Pegvisomant is an antagonist of GH receptor with a good efficacy. It can be used alone or in association with somatostatin analog or cabergoline if acromegaly is not controlled with somatostatin analog alone. The efficacy in real life is around 75% in acromegaly and 50% for gigantism. Indeed, pegvisomant can be used in the second medical stage after somatostatin analog.

Author details

Claire Briet*, Valentine Suteau and Patrice Rodien

*Address all correspondence to: claire.briet@chu-angers.fr

Endocrinology, Diabetology and Nutrition Department, INSERM U1083, Institut Mitovasc, CHU, Angers, France

References

[1] Abdel-Meguid SS, Shieh HS, Smith WW, Dayringer HE, Violand BN, Bentle LA. Three-dimensional structure of a genetically engineered variant of porcine growth hormone. Proceedings of the National Academy of Sciences of the United States of America. 1987;**84**:6434-6437

[2] Hara K, Hsu Chen CJ, Sonenberg M. Recombination of the biologically active peptides from a tryptic digest of bovine growth hormone. Biochemistry. 1978;**17**:550-556

[3] Chen WY, Wight DC, Wagner TE, Kopchick JJ. Expression of a mutated bovine growth hormone gene suppresses growth of transgenic mice. Proceedings of the National Academy of Sciences of the United States of America. 1990;**87**:5061-5065

[4] de Vos AM, Ultsch M, Kossiakoff AA. Human growth hormone and extracellular domain of its receptor: Crystal structure of the complex. Science. 1992;**255**:306-312

[5] Cunningham BC, Wells JA. Rational design of receptor-specific variants of human growth hormone. Proceedings of the National Academy of Sciences of the United States of America. 1991;**88**:3407-3411

[6] Ross RJ, Leung KC, Maamra M, Bennett W, Doyle N, Waters MJ, et al. Binding and functional studies with the growth hormone receptor antagonist, B2036-PEG (pegvisomant), reveal effects of pegylation and evidence that it binds to a receptor dimer. The Journal of Clinical Endocrinology and Metabolism. 2001;**86**:1716-1723

[7] Yang N, Langenheim JF, Wang X, Jiang J, Chen WY, Frank SJ. Activation of growth hormone receptors by growth hormone and growth hormone antagonist dimers: Insights into receptor triggering. Molecular Endocrinology. 2008;**22**:978-988

[8] Lan H, Li W, Li R, Zheng X, Luo G. Endocytosis and degradation of Pegvisomant and a potential new mechanism that inhibits the nuclear translocation of GHR. The Journal of Clinical Endocrinology and Metabolism. 2019;**104**:1887-1899

[9] Thorner MO, Strasburger CJ, Wu Z, Straume M, Bidlingmaier M, Pezzoli SS, et al. Growth hormone (GH) receptor blockade with a PEG-modified GH (B2036-PEG) lowers serum insulin-like growth factor-I but does not acutely stimulate serum GH. The Journal of Clinical Endocrinology and Metabolism. 1999;**84**:2098-2103

[10] van der Lely AJ, Lamberts S, Barkan A, Panadya N, Besser GM, Trainer PJ, et al. A six week, double blind, placebo controlled study of a growth hormone antagonist, B2036-PEG (Trovert) in acromegalic patients. In: Program of the 80th Annual Meeting of the Endocrine Society, New Orleans, LA. 1998. p. 57

[11] Trainer PJ, Drake WM, Katznelson L, Freda PU, Herman-Bonert V, van der Lely AJ, et al. Treatment of acromegaly with the growth hormone-receptor antagonist pegvisomant. The New England Journal of Medicine. 2000;**342**:1171-1177

[12] van der Lely AJ, Hutson RK, Trainer PJ, Besser GM, Barkan AL, Katznelson L, et al. Long-term treatment of acromegaly with pegvisomant, a growth hormone receptor antagonist. Lancet. 2001;**358**:1754-1759

[13] Buchfelder M, van der Lely AJ, Biller BMK, Webb SM, Brue T, Strasburger CJ, et al. Long-term treatment with pegvisomant: Observations from 2090 acromegaly patients in ACROSTUDY. European Journal of Endocrinology. 2018;**179**:419-427

[14] Boguszewski CL, Huayllas MKP, Vilar L, Naves LA, Ribeiro-Oliveira Junior A, Soares BS, et al. Brazilian multicenter study on pegvisomant treatment in acromegaly. Archives of Endocrinology and Metabolism. 2019;**63**:328-336

[15] Leonart LP, Tonin FS, Ferreira VL, Fernandez-Llimos F, Pontarolo R. Effectiveness and safety of pegvisomant: A systematic review and meta-analysis of observational longitudinal studies. Endocrine. 2019;**63**:18-26

[16] Puglisi S, Spagnolo F, Ragonese M, Cannavo S, Ferrau F. First report on persistent remission of acromegaly after withdrawal of long-term pegvisomant monotherapy. Growth Hormone & IGF Research. 2019;**45**:17-19

[17] Camara R, Venegas E, Garcia-Arnes JA, Cordido F, Aller J, Samaniego ML, et al. Treatment adherence to pegvisomant in patients with acromegaly in Spain: PEGASO study. Pituitary. 2019;**22**:137-145

[18] Garcia WR, Cortes HT, Romero AF. Pituitary gigantism: A case series from hospital de San Jose (Bogota, Colombia). Archives of Endocrinology and Metabolism. 2019;**63**:385-393

[19] Rostomyan L, Daly AF, Petrossians P, Nachev E, Lila AR, et al. Beckers A 2015 Clinical and genetic characterization of pituitary gigantism: An international collaborative study in 208 patients. Endocrine-Related Cancer 22:745-757

[20] Katznelson L, Laws ER Jr, Melmed S, Molitch ME, Murad MH, Utz A, et al. Acromegaly: An endocrine society clinical practice guideline. The Journal of Clinical Endocrinology and Metabolism. 2014;**99**:3933-3951

[21] Sandret L, Maison P, Chanson P. Place of cabergoline in acromegaly: A meta-analysis. The Journal of Clinical Endocrinology and Metabolism. 2011;**96**:1327-1335

[22] Kuhn E, Chanson P. Cabergoline in acromegaly. Pituitary. 2017;**20**:121-128

[23] Lamberts SWJ, Hofland LJ. Anniversary review: Octreotide, 40 years later. European Journal of Endocrinology. 2019;**181**:R173-R183

[24] Shimon I, Adnan Z, Gorshtein A, Baraf L, Saba Khazen N, Gershinsky M, et al. Efficacy and safety of long-acting pasireotide in patients with somatostatin-resistant acromegaly: A multicenter study. Endocrine. 2018;**62**:448-455

[25] Giustina A, Barkan A, Beckers A, Biermasz N, Biller BMK, Boguszewski C, et al. A consensus on the diagnosis and treatment of acromegaly comorbidities: An update. The Journal of Clinical Endocrinology and Metabolism. 2019

[26] Melmed S, Bronstein MD, Chanson P, Klibanski A, Casanueva FF, Wass JAH, et al. A consensus statement on acromegaly therapeutic outcomes. Nature Reviews. Endocrinology. 2018;**14**:552-561

[27] Elbaum M, Mizera L, Bolanowski M. The real costs of acromegaly: Analysis of different therapies. Endokrynologia Polska. 2019;**70**:74-85

[28] Trainer PJ, Ezzat S, D'Souza GA, Layton G, Strasburger CJ. A randomized, controlled, multicentre trial comparing pegvisomant alone with combination therapy of pegvisomant and long-acting octreotide in patients with acromegaly. Clinical Endocrinology. 2009;**71**:549-557

[29] Neggers SJ, Franck SE, de Rooij FW, Dallenga AH, Poublon RM, Feelders RA, et al. Long-term efficacy and safety of pegvisomant in combination with long-acting somatostatin analogs in acromegaly. The Journal of Clinical Endocrinology and Metabolism. 2014;**99**:3644-3652

[30] Giustina A, Bevan JS, Bronstein MD, Casanueva FF, Chanson P, Petersenn S, et al. SAGIT(R): Clinician-reported outcome instrument for managing acromegaly in clinical practice-development and results from a pilot study. Pituitary. 2016;**19**:39-49

[31] van der Lely AJ, Gomez R, Pleil A, Badia X, Brue T, Buchfelder M, Burman P, Clemmons D, Ghigo E, Jorgensen JOL, Luger A, van der Lans-Bussemaker J, Webb SM, Strasburger CJ 2017 Development of ACRODAT((R)), a new software medical device to assess disease activity in patients with acromegaly. Pituitary 20:692-701

[32] Webb SM, Badia X, Surinach NL, Spanish AcroQol Study Group. Validity and clinical applicability of the acromegaly quality of life questionnaire, AcroQoL: A 6-month prospective study. European Journal of Endocrinology. 2006;**155**:269-277

[33] Basavilbaso NXG, Ballarino MC, Bruera D, Bruno OD, Chervin AB, Danilowicz K, et al. Pegvisomant in acromegaly: A multicenter real-life study in Argentina. Arch Endocrinol Metab. 2019;**63**:320-327

[34] Barkan AL, Burman P, Clemmons DR, Drake WM, Gagel RF, Harris PE, et al. Glucose homeostasis and safety in patients with acromegaly converted from long-acting octreotide to pegvisomant. The Journal of Clinical Endocrinology and Metabolism. 2005;**90**: 5684-5691

[35] Brue T, Lindberg A, Jan van der Lely A, Akerblad AC, Koltowska-Haggstrom M, Gomez R, et al. Diabetes in patients with acromegaly treated with pegvisomant: Observations from acrostudy. Endocrine. 2019;**63**:563-572

[36] Feola T, Cozzolino A, Simonelli I, Sbardella E, Pozza C, Giannetta E, et al. Pegvisomant improves glucose metabolism in acromegaly: A meta-analysis of prospective interventional studies. The Journal of Clinical Endocrinology and Metabolism. 2019;**104**:2892-2902

[37] Freda PU, Gordon MB, Kelepouris N, Jonsson P, Koltowska-Haggstrom M, van der Lely AJ. Long-term treatment with pegvisomant as monotherapy in patients with acromegaly: Experience from ACROSTUDY. Endocrine Practice. 2015;**21**:264-274

[38] Chiloiro S, Mormando M, Bianchi A, Giampietro A, Milardi D, Bima C, et al. Prevalence of morphometric vertebral fractures in "difficult" patients with acromegaly with different biochemical outcomes after multimodal treatment. Endocrine. 2018;**59**:449-453

[39] Chiloiro S, Antonella G, Frara S, Bima C, Donfrancesco F, Maya FC, et al. Effects of pegvisomant and pasireotide LAR on vertebral fractures in acromegaly resistant to

first-generation SRLs. Journal of Clinical Endocrinology and Metabolism. 2019. pii: dgz054

[40] Chiloiro S, Mazziotti G, Giampietro A, Bianchi A, Frara S, Mormando M, et al. Effects of pegvisomant and somatostatin receptor ligands on incidence of vertebral fractures in patients with acromegaly. Pituitary. 2018;**21**:302-308

Chapter 8

Colorectal Neoplasm in Acromegaly: Epidemiology and Underlying Mechanisms

Masaaki Yamamoto and Yutaka Takahashi

Additional information is available at the end of the chapter

http://dx.doi.org/10.5772/intechopen.91336

Abstract

Acromegaly is characterized by autonomous growth hormone (GH) secretion from the pituitary somatotroph adenoma and increased levels of serum insulin-like growth factor I (IGF-I). These conditions are associated with increased morbidity and mortality due to metabolic conditions, cardiovascular diseases, and malignant neoplasms. Among neoplasms, while colorectal neoplasms are a well-known comorbidity in patients with acromegaly, the prevalence of colorectal benign or malignant tumors varies among studies. Although several underlying mechanisms have been proposed, recent studies have unveiled new insights into tumorigenesis. This review focused on the epidemiological studies of colorectal neoplasm in acromegaly and recent advances in the elucidation of the underlying mechanisms.

Keywords: acromegaly, colon polyp, colon cancer, GH, IGF-I

1. Introduction

Acromegaly is characterized by excess levels of insulin-like growth factor I (IGF-I) derived from autonomous growth hormone (GH) secretion from the pituitary somatotroph adenoma, which results in acral enlargement, coarse facial features, and visceromegaly [1, 2]. Even worse, acromegalic patients exhibit a shorter life span than healthy subjects owing to various comorbidities such as diabetes; hypertension; and cardiovascular, cerebrovascular, and respiratory diseases [1]. Malignant neoplasms in several organs including the thyroid, breast, prostate, pancreas, and digestive tract are also widely recognized as representative complications [1, 3, 4]. Even among those, patients with acromegaly are well known to have a significantly higher prevalence of colon neoplasms than the general population. Recent evidence suggests

IntechOpen

© 2020 The Author(s). Licensee IntechOpen. This chapter is distributed under the terms of the Creative Commons Attribution License (http://creativecommons.org/licenses/by/3.0), which permits unrestricted use, distribution, and reproduction in any medium, provided the original work is properly cited.

that even benign neoplasms such as adenoma and hyperplasia may have the potential to develop into malignant adenocarcinoma, which potentially affects the prognosis of acromegalic patients [5–7]. Recent guidelines recommend that while acromegalic patients are necessary to undergo colonoscopy regularly, they often face difficulties throughout colonoscopy intubation owing to distinctive features of acromegaly such as elongation of the colon [8]. Recently, the molecular mechanism behind colon tumorigenesis associated with the GH-IGF-I excess has been elucidated. In this chapter, we review the epidemiological evidence, protocol of follow-up colonoscopy, and underlying mechanism of GH/IGF-I-associated colon tumorigenesis in patients with acromegaly.

2. Epidemiology in colorectal neoplasms in acromegaly

Klein et al. first demonstrated an increased prevalence of colon polyps in patients with acromegaly in 1982, reporting a prevalence of colorectal adenomatous polyps of approximately 30% in 17 patients with acromegaly [9]. Several subsequent reports also showed that colonic neoplasms were more frequently observed in 47% of patients with acromegaly, compared to the control with colonic lesions in 40% of asymptomatic males >50 years [10]. A cohort study identified 1041 male patients as having acromegaly from over 4 million men from the database of the United States Veterans Administration, which revealed a prevalence of acromegaly to be 277 cases/million [11]. In this study, 13 acromegalic patients had colonic cancer, which indicates a significantly higher prevalence than in the control group (SIR: 3.1; 95% CI 1.7–5.1) [11]. The UK registry of acromegaly diagnosed 16 patients as having colorectal cancer from a total of 1239 patients with acromegaly. Although this study did not show any significant change in the frequency of colorectal carcinoma compared to healthy subjects, the mortality rate of colon cancer was higher even though the overall mortality rate due to cancer was not increased [4]. An investigation of the incidence of cancer in 1643 hospitalized acromegalic patients in North Europe was performed, and the estimated standardized incidence ratio (SIR) was 2.6 (95% confidence interval [CI] 1.6–3.8) for overall colorectal cancer and 2.5 (95% CI 1.3–4.2) for rectal carcinoma [12]. Terzolo et al. performed colonoscopy to screen for colorectal tumors in 235 patients with acromegaly and compared the prevalence of colorectal tumors in this cohort with the prevalence in a control population who had no past and family history of colonic disease. Patients with acromegaly exhibited a higher prevalence of colon adenomas (acromegaly; 23.4% vs. control; 14.6%; $P = 0.001$), hyperplastic polyps (19.1% vs. 9.4%; $P = 0.003$), and cancer (4.3% vs. 0.9%; $P = 0.036$) [13]. The risk factor for colon cancer in acromegaly was young age, whereas there was no association between the prevalence of colon neoplasms and serum IGF-1 levels or disease duration [13]. Delhougne et al. reported similar results of acromegalic patients showing an increased prevalence of adenomatous (22.3% vs. 8%; $P = 0.0024$) and hyperplastic polyps (24.3% vs. 4.4%; $P < 0.001$) compared to a control group [14]. In particular, younger people (younger than 55 years old) and men had a higher prevalence of adenomatous polyp than those in the control group (20.3% vs. 3.0%; $P < 0.0026$) [14]. Our recent study revealed that 57 Japanese acromegalic patients also exhibited a higher prevalence of colon adenomas (31.6% vs. 2.5%; $P < 0.0001$) and hyperplastic polyps (38.6% vs. 6.7%; $P < 0.0001$) than the historical control group with irritable bowel syndrome [15].

Furthermore, colon cancer in patients with acromegaly exhibited an increased odds ratio of 14.5 (95% CI 5.8–23.3) compared to that in the general Japanese population [15].

Thus, numerous studies documented evidence regarding risk of colorectal tumors in acromegalic patients, and several meta-analyses have demonstrated an increased prevalence of colorectal tumors including benign polyps and carcinomas. A German review meta-analyzed 9 eligible papers with strict inclusion criteria from 106 studies. As benign polyps, the pooled ORs with 95% CI of hyperplastic polyps and colon adenomas were 3.7 (95% CI; 2.6–5.3) and 2.5 (95% CI; 1.9–3.4), respectively. In terms of colon cancer, the pooled OR with 95% CI was 4.4 (1.5–12.4) [16]. The second study meta-analyzed 14 papers to determine the incidence of colorectal cancer [17]. After exclusion criteria was <10 expected cases, standardized incidence ratios (SIRs) were obtained from eight studies and the pooled SIR was 2.6 (95% CI; 1.7–4.0), which demonstrated an increased prevalence of colorectal cancer [18]. While the prevalence of colorectal cancer in female was significantly increased (SIR 1.86; 95% CI, 1.06–3.28 $P = 0.03$), male patients had no change (SIR 1.44; 95% CI, 0.72–2.88 $P = 0.31$) [17]. An analysis of patients with acromegaly including male and female patients revealed that the SIR of colorectal cancer with 95% CI was significantly elevated (SIR 1.67; 95% CI, 1.07–2.58, P = 0.022) [17]. Taken together, these meta-analyses demonstrated an increased risk of colorectal cancer in patients with acromegaly. There was a large variance in SIRs among studies from 1.4 [4] to 18.2 [3] and the difference in SIRs was observed depends on single center trials (SIR 7.3) and multicenter or population-based trials (SIR 2.0 and 2.2, respectively). In addition, two meta-analyses demonstrated that Japanese cohorts exhibited obviously higher prevalence of colorectal cancer in acromegalic patients than in other countries, suggesting that there may be an ethnic difference [16, 18].

3. Follow-up colonoscopy based on guidelines

Although some studies described the frequency of colonoscopy for the follow-up in patients with acromegaly, there is still controversy on the appropriate follow-up [13, 19, 20]. The guidelines in 2002 recommended that colonoscopy should be performed every 3–5 years considering the past history of colon neoplasms and family history [21]. The next revision in 2009 suggested that colonoscopy should be performed at least once upon diagnosis in all patients with acromegaly. If colon polyps were detected in patients with acromegaly at the first screening, they should be carefully followed up based on the guidelines of screening and surveillance for general colorectal cancer [22–24]. However, several groups still appealed the importance of repeated colonoscopy on a regular basis for acromegalic patients [25–27]. Dworakowska et al. reported that patients who were diagnosed as having adenomatous polyp at first screening had a higher risk of developing a new lesion at the subsequent follow-up colonoscopy. Additionally, patients with poor IGF-I control had a 7.5-fold higher risk of a subsequent adenoma even if patients had a normal colon at the first screening [20].

The British Society of Gastroenterology and the Association of Coloproctology for Great Britain and Ireland in 2010 classified acromegalic patients as having a moderate to high risk of colorectal cancer on the update of the 2002 guidance, which suggested performing colonoscopy screening in those 40 years of age or older on a regular basis [28]. The frequency of repeat colonoscopy should be modified depending on the conditions of the initial screening and the activity of acromegaly. If the initial screening test showed negative results and IGF-I level was within normal range, the next colonoscopy will be scheduled 5–10 years later. When adenomatous polyps were detected at initial screening or higher IGF-I levels were noted, follow-up colonoscopy should be performed every 3 years [28]. The medical guidelines of the American Association of Clinical Endocrinologists (2011) and the Acromegaly Consensus Group (2013) state a similar recommendation that acromegalic patients should undergo initial colonoscopy at the time of diagnosis. If persistently elevated IGF-I level, abnormal findings by colonoscopy, or a family history of colon cancer is noted, follow-up colonoscopy should be performed more frequently. If not, a follow-up colonoscopy should be recommended every 10 years [29, 30].

Although current recommendations for surveillance colonoscopy in acromegaly may differ slightly among each study, collectively, it is deemed necessary to perform follow-up colonoscopy for cases with poor control of IGF-I and adenomatous polyps at least every 5 years according to five independent statements [20, 28, 29, 31]. Although an updated consensus from the Acromegaly Consensus Group in 2019 still recommends screening by colonoscopy at the time of diagnosis, they toned down the recommendation in terms of follow-up colonoscopy on a regular basis because there is no evidence linking screening frequency to colon cancer mortality rates [32, 33]. As acromegalic patients live longer than before owing to the improvement of biochemical control by advances in the treatment strategy, aging seems to be a more reliable indicator of cancer in patients with acromegaly than GH/IGF-I excess [34].

4. Underlying mechanism of colon neoplasm in acromegaly

4.1. GH signal

Secreted GH interacts with the GH receptor (GHR) that belongs to the class I cytokine receptor family, which is mainly expressed in the liver, fat, and muscle [35]. Consequently, phosphorylated GHR induces janus kinase 2 (JAK2) phosphorylation, which results in tyrosine phosphorylation of STAT5 (signal transducer and activator of transcription 5). STAT5 is the physiologically essential transcription factor for GH-dependent body growth, lipid metabolism, and sex-specific gene expression [36]. Recent studies have revealed that STAT5 plays an important role in tumorigenesis, especially cell proliferation and exertion of the anti-apoptotic property [37]. The phosphorylated STAT5 is associated with the development of malignant neoplasms including malignant prostate neoplasms, malignant breast neoplasms, and leukemia [37–39]. In colorectal cancer, the expression level of STAT5B is higher than in the normal colon tissue, and also correlates with the TNM stage [40]. Furthermore, phosphorylated STAT5 in colon adenocarcinomas is associated with a poor prognosis [41]. The phosphorylation of STAT5 is suppressed by suppressor of cytokine signaling-2 (SOCS2) in the GH signaling pathway [42]. A previous paper reported that SOCS2-knockout exhibited the development of hyperplastic mucosa and polyps in bovine GH-transgenic mice [43] Furthermore, d3GHR polymorphism caused the signaling enhancement, which resulted in increasing the risk of colon adenoma regardless of circulating IGF-I concentration compared to intact GHR in acromegalic patients [44]. Recently, we reported that the GH area under the curve in the oral glucose tolerance test exhibited higher prevalence in colon cancer patients than in colonic benign tumor patients [15]. These data suggest the significance of excessive GH signaling in the development of epithelium-adenoma-carcinoma, independent of IGF-I signaling [45].

4.2. IGF-I signal

Bowel enlargement in acromegalic patients is observed associated with accumulative excessive GH and IGF-I [46–48]. Enhanced proliferation of colonic epithelial cells and reduced apoptosis of the colonic mucosa were observed in patients with acromegaly [47, 49]. Interestingly, an increased proliferation rate of colonic epithelium cells was correlated with circulating IGF1 levels [50]. IGF-I receptor knockout mice exhibited a decreased cell proliferation and increased apoptosis [1]. The IGF-I/IGF-IR system also plays an important role in the promotion of cell adhesion, migration, and tumor microenvironment including the angiogenesis in the tumor [51]. The IGF-IR mRNA expression level in the colon cancer tissue was associated with paracrine/autocrine effects [1]. Even in those with normal IGF-I levels, there was a positive association between circulating IGF-I levels and the risk of colorectal cancer in a meta-analysis of 19 epidemiological studies [52]. However, several previous studies suggested that the classification based on the type of colorectal neoplasms or with/without colorectal neoplasms did not correlate with serum IGF-I levels [13, 15, 53, 54]. Taken together, elevated levels of serum IGF-I may also involve colorectal tumorigenesis, but it still needs further investigation.

4.3. Local GH action in the colon

In terms of direct action of GH as a novel insight, it has recently been reported that locally expressed GH in the colon is a precursor to colon cancer. Excessive GH leads to cell survival with downregulation of tumor suppressor genes such as p53 and APC, which results in neoplastic colon growth [55]. GH suppressed DNA damage response (DDR) by inhibiting phosphorylated ataxia telangiectasia mutated (ATM), checkpoint kinase 2 (Chk2), and p53. They also elucidated that GH significantly increased unrepaired DNA damage in colon epithelial cells, and colon cancer cell lines of xenografted mice with GH overexpression exhibited more metastases compared to colon cancer cell lines of control mice [56], and these mechanisms were observed independent of IGF-I action [57].

5. Underlying mechanism of hyperplastic polyp in acromegaly

As mentioned above, various mechanisms are involved in tumorigenesis of colorectal neoplasms. These mechanisms can account for the tumorigenesis of colorectal adenomatous polyps or adenocarcinomas, but not hyperplastic polyps. As a noteworthy fact, hyperplastic polyps are basically considered as benign neoplasms, while colorectal adenoma is widely recognized as pre-malignant conditions based on the presence of the adenoma-carcinoma sequence. Indeed, hyperplastic polyps are described by a superficial serrated architecture and variably elongated crypts with proliferation confined to the lower portion of the crypt [58]. However, *k-ras* or *BRAF* mutations and microsatellite instability, which cause the malignant colorectal tumors, are detected in hyperplastic polyps [6]. In this aspect, hyperplastic polyps may need to be carefully diagnosed with histological examination in acromegaly. Acromegalic patients exhibited accelerated mucosal proliferation in the colon tissue compared to normal subjects [47, 59], which might involve in an increased prevalence of hyperplastic polyps. Further investigation is needed to elucidate the potential risk and underlying mechanism of the development of hyperplastic polyps in acromegaly.

6. Conclusion

Colorectal neoplasm, especially adenocarcinoma, is a life-threatening comorbidity of acromegaly. Accumulating data clearly demonstrate the increased prevalence of colorectal polyps and cancer in patients with acromegaly even among different races and countries. Although the appropriate follow-up protocol of colonoscopy remains controversial, different guidelines state that cases with poor control IGF-I and adenomatous polyps should be classified as having a high risk of colon cancer. In terms of molecular mechanisms, both GH and IGF-I are implicated in colon cancer development.

Author details

Masaaki Yamamoto[1] and Yutaka Takahashi[2*]

*Address all correspondence to: takahash@med.kobe-u.ac.jp

1 Division of Diabetes and Endocrinology, Kobe University Hospital, Kobe, Japan

2 Division of Diabetes and Endocrinology, Kobe University Graduate School of Medicine, Kobe, Japan

References

[1] Colao A et al. Systemic complications of acromegaly: Epidemiology, pathogenesis, and management. Endocrine Reviews. 2004;**25**(1):102-152

[2] Melmed S. Acromegaly pathogenesis and treatment. The Journal of Clinical Investigation. 2009;**119**(11):3189-3202

[3] Kurimoto M et al. The prevalence of benign and malignant tumors in patients with acromegaly at a single institute. Endocrine Journal. 2008;**55**(1):67-71

[4] Orme SM et al. Mortality and cancer incidence in acromegaly: A retrospective cohort study. The Journal of Clinical Endocrinology and Metabolism. 1998;**83**(8):2730-2734

[5] Jass JR et al. Emerging concepts in colorectal neoplasia. Gastroenterology. 2002;**123**(3): 862-876

[6] Snover DC et al. Serrated polyps of the large intestine: A morphologic and molecular review of an evolving concept. American Journal of Clinical Pathology. 2005;**124**(3):380-391

[7] Torlakovic E et al. Morphologic reappraisal of serrated colorectal polyps. The American Journal of Surgical Pathology. 2003;**27**(1):65-81

[8] Iwamuro M et al. Colonoscopy examination requires a longer time in patients with acromegaly than in other individuals. Endocrine Journal. 2018;**65**(2):151-157

[9] Klein I et al. Colonic polyps in patients with acromegaly. Annals of Internal Medicine. 1982;**97**(1):27-30

[10] Melmed S. Acromegaly and cancer: Not a problem? The Journal of Clinical Endocrinology and Metabolism. 2001;**86**(7):2929-2934

[11] Ron E et al. Acromegaly and gastrointestinal cancer. Cancer. 1991;**68**(8):1673-1677

[12] Baris D et al. Acromegaly and cancer risk: A cohort study in Sweden and Denmark. Cancer Causes & Control. 2002;**13**(5):395-400

[13] Terzolo M et al. Colonoscopic screening and follow-up in patients with acromegaly: A multicenter study in Italy. The Journal of Clinical Endocrinology and Metabolism. 2005;**90**(1):84-90

[14] Delhougne B et al. The prevalence of colonic polyps in acromegaly: A colonoscopic and pathological study in 103 patients. The Journal of Clinical Endocrinology and Metabolism. 1995;**80**(11):3223-3226

[15] Yamamoto M et al. The prevalence and associated factors of colorectal neoplasms in acromegaly: A single center based study. Pituitary. 2015;**18**(3):343-351

[16] Rokkas T et al. Risk of colorectal neoplasm in patients with acromegaly: A meta-analysis. World Journal of Gastroenterology. 2008;**14**(22):3484-3489

[17] Terzolo M et al. Acromegaly is associated with increased cancer risk: A survey in Italy. Endocrine-Related Cancer. 2017;**24**(9):495-504

[18] Dal J et al. Cancer incidence in patients with acromegaly: A cohort study and meta-analysis of the literature. The Journal of Clinical Endocrinology and Metabolism. 2018;**103**(6): 2182-2188

[19] Parolin M et al. Guidelines versus real life practice: The case of colonoscopy in acromegaly. Pituitary. 2018;**21**(1):16-24

[20] Dworakowska D et al. Repeated colonoscopic screening of patients with acromegaly: 15-year experience identifies those at risk of new colonic neoplasia and allows for effective screening guidelines. European Journal of Endocrinology. 2010;**163**(1):21-28

[21] Melmed S et al. Guidelines for acromegaly management. The Journal of Clinical Endocrinology and Metabolism. 2002;**87**(9):4054-4058

[22] Melmed S et al. Guidelines for acromegaly management: An update. The Journal of Clinical Endocrinology and Metabolism. 2009;**94**(5):1509-1517

[23] Sung JJ et al. Asia Pacific consensus recommendations for colorectal cancer screening. Gut. 2008;**57**(8):1166-1176

[24] Levin B et al. Screening and surveillance for the early detection of colorectal cancer and adenomatous polyps, 2008: A joint guideline from the American Cancer Society, the US multi-society task force on colorectal Cancer, and the American College of Radiology. Gastroenterology. 2008;**134**(5):1570-1595

[25] Jenkins PJ et al. Insulin-like growth factor I and the development of colorectal neoplasia in acromegaly. The Journal of Clinical Endocrinology and Metabolism. 2000;**85**(9):3218-3221

[26] Jenkins PJ, Fairclough PD. Colorectal neoplasia in acromegaly. Clinical Endocrinology. 2001;**55**(6):727-729

[27] Perry I, Stewart PM, Kane K. Colorectal screening guidelines in acromegaly. Gut. 2003;**52**(9):1387. author reply 1387

[28] Cairns SR et al. Guidelines for colorectal cancer screening and surveillance in moderate and high risk groups (update from 2002). Gut. 2010;**59**(5):666-689

[29] Melmed S et al. A consensus on the diagnosis and treatment of acromegaly complications. Pituitary. 2013;**16**(3):294-302

[30] Katznelson L et al. American Association of Clinical Endocrinologists medical guidelines for clinical practice for the diagnosis and treatment of acromegaly—2011 update. Endocrine Practice. 2011;**17**(Suppl 4):1-44

[31] Giustina A et al. Expert consensus document: A consensus on the medical treatment of acromegaly. Nature Reviews. Endocrinology. 2014;**10**(4):243-248

[32] Lois K et al. The role of colonoscopic screening in acromegaly revisited: Review of current literature and practice guidelines. Pituitary. 2015;**18**(4):568-574

[33] Giustina A et al. A consensus on the diagnosis and treatment of acromegaly comorbidities: An update. The Journal of Clinical Endocrinology and Metabolism. 2019. (in press)

[34] Bolfi F et al. Mortality in acromegaly decreased in the last decade: A systematic review and meta-analysis. European Journal of Endocrinology. 2018;**179**(1):59-71

[35] Brown RJ et al. Model for growth hormone receptor activation based on subunit rotation within a receptor dimer. Nature Structural & Molecular Biology. 2005;**12**(9):814-821

[36] Lanning NJ, Carter-Su C. Recent advances in growth hormone signaling. Reviews in Endocrine & Metabolic Disorders. 2006;**7**(4):225-235

[37] Ferbeyre G, Moriggl R. The role of Stat5 transcription factors as tumor suppressors or oncogenes. Biochimica et Biophysica Acta. 2011;**1815**(1):104-114

[38] Nevalainen MT et al. Signal transducer and activator of transcription-5 activation and breast cancer prognosis. Journal of Clinical Oncology. 2004;**22**(11):2053-2060

[39] Tan SH, Nevalainen MT. Signal transducer and activator of transcription 5A/B in prostate and breast cancers. Endocrine-Related Cancer. 2008;**15**(2):367-390

[40] Du W et al. STAT5 isoforms regulate colorectal cancer cell apoptosis via reduction of mitochondrial membrane potential and generation of reactive oxygen species. Journal of Cellular Physiology. 2012;**227**(6):2421-2429

[41] Mao YL et al. Phospho-STAT5 expression is associated with poor prognosis of human colonic adenocarcinoma. Pathology Oncology Research. 2011;**17**(2):333-339

[42] Favre H et al. Dual effects of suppressor of cytokine signaling (SOCS-2) on growth hormone signal transduction. FEBS Letters. 1999;**453**(1-2):63-66

[43] Michaylira CZ et al. Haplotype insufficiency for suppressor of cytokine signaling-2 enhances intestinal growth and promotes polyp formation in growth hormone-transgenic mice. Endocrinology. 2006;**147**(4):1632-1641

[44] Wassenaar MJ et al. Acromegaly is associated with an increased prevalence of colonic diverticula: A case-control study. The Journal of Clinical Endocrinology and Metabolism. 2010;**95**(5):2073-2079

[45] Vogelstein B et al. Genetic alterations during colorectal-tumor development. The New England Journal of Medicine. 1988;**319**(9):525-532

[46] Reinmuth N et al. Blockade of insulin-like growth factor I receptor function inhibits growth and angiogenesis of colon cancer. Clinical Cancer Research. 2002;**8**(10):3259-3269

[47] Cats A et al. Increased epithelial cell proliferation in the colon of patients with acromegaly. Cancer Research. 1996;**56**(3):523-526

[48] Ewton DZ et al. Insulin-like growth factor-I has a biphasic effect on colon carcinoma cells through transient inactivation of forkhead1, initially mitogenic, then mediating growth arrest and differentiation. International Journal of Cancer. 2002;**98**(5):665-673

[49] Bogazzi F et al. Apoptosis is reduced in the colonic mucosa of patients with acromegaly. Clinical Endocrinology. 2005;**63**(6):683-688

[50] Gonzalez B et al. The prevalence of colonic polyps in patients with acromegaly: A case-control, nested in a cohort colonoscopic study. Endocrine Practice. 2017;**23**(5):594-599

[51] Baserga R. The contradictions of the insulin-like growth factor 1 receptor. Oncogene. 2000;**19**(49):5574-5581

[52] Chi F et al. Circulation insulin-like growth factor peptides and colorectal cancer risk: An updated systematic review and meta-analysis. Molecular Biology Reports. 2013;**40**(5):3583-3590

[53] Colao A et al. The association of fasting insulin concentrations and colonic neoplasms in acromegaly: A colonoscopy-based study in 210 patients. The Journal of Clinical Endocrinology and Metabolism. 2007;**92**(10):3854-3860

[54] Renehan AG et al. The prevalence and characteristics of colorectal neoplasia in acromegaly. The Journal of Clinical Endocrinology and Metabolism. 2000;**85**(9):3417-3424

[55] Chesnokova V et al. Growth hormone is permissive for neoplastic colon growth. Proceedings of the National Academy of Sciences of the United States of America. 2016; **113**(23):E3250-E3259

[56] Chesnokova V et al. Excess growth hormone suppresses DNA damage repair in epithelial cells. JCI Insight. 2019;**4**(3):e125762

[57] Chesnokova V et al. Growth hormone induces Colon DNA damage independent of IGF-1. Endocrinology. 2019;**160**(6):1439-1447

[58] Williams GT. Metaplastic (hyperplastic) polyps of the large bowel: Benign neoplasms after all? Gut. 1997;**40**(5):691-692

[59] Jenkins PJ. Acromegaly and colon cancer. Growth Hormone & IGF Research. 2000;**10** (Suppl A):S35-S36

Chapter 9

The Surgical Management of Acromegaly

John L. Kilgallon and Edward R. Laws

Additional information is available at the end of the chapter

http://dx.doi.org/10.5772/intechopen.91430

Abstract

Acromegaly is the condition produced by one of the benign tumors of the pituitary gland. These tumors produce a variety of disorders affecting many parts of the body, producing side effects related to abnormal hormone function. The dramatic appearance of the acromegalic giant has attracted attention over the ages. This chapter summarizes the history of the recognition and ultimate diagnosis of acromegaly. The biological and physiological elements are described. The methods of diagnosis and management are elaborated. Although the focus of the chapter is on the surgical approach for treatment, alternative strategies are also discussed, along with the outcomes of management for patients and the restoration of quality of life as a primary goal.

Keywords: acromegaly, gigantism, growth hormone, pituitary surgery, endoscopic surgery

1. Introduction

By 1800, the existence of human "giants" had been established through legends and stories for centuries. Up to that point, the story of "O'Brien the Irish Giant" was one of the most intriguing. Charles Byrne, O'Brien's given name, was born in Ireland in 1761 and died in London in 1783 at the age of 22 [1]. During the course of his short life, his legend grew to the level of national fame in Great Britain and continued after he died. Byrne's notoriety stemmed from his terrific stature, alleged at the time to be 8 feet 4 inches. In truth, he stood at about 7 feet and 7 inches tall, still towering over the spectators who paid to see him. As a teenager, Byrne left Ireland for Britain, where he intended to make a name for himself by displaying his body and charging people for the chance to come see him. Sadly, Byrne's career would end tragically one night at a pub where he was robbed of his life's earnings, as much as £700. He died shortly

IntechOpen

© 2020 The Author(s). Licensee IntechOpen. This chapter is distributed under the terms of the Creative Commons Attribution License (http://creativecommons.org/licenses/by/3.0), which permits unrestricted use, distribution, and reproduction in any medium, provided the original work is properly cited. (cc) BY

thereafter. Upon his death, a competition began among medical professionals to secure the rights to his corpse, in some cases for the purpose of scientific research, in others out of curiosity and greed. Byrne had foreseen this outcome and had made it known that he did not wish for anyone to dissect his body after he died, requesting that he be buried at sea [1]. This did not stop the pursuit of Byrne's body, and it was the infamous John Hunter who "managed to surreptitiously procure Byrne's corpse from a dishonest person among Byrne's companions for a large sum, quoted at £500." [1] Instead of examining Byrne's pituitary fossa, Hunter was actually seeking Byrne's body as a collector's item and decided to display the man's skeleton in his museum [2]. For over a century, his skull would remain unexamined; in the meantime, the medical world's understanding of gigantism and acromegaly would grow exponentially.

In 1864, the Italian neurologist Andre Verga first documented a patient who displayed symptoms of a certain affliction which he named "prosopectasia," or a widening of the face, a common sign of the disease we now call acromegaly [3] (**Figure 1**).

That same year, Verga also became one of the earliest investigators to report an acromegalic subject with a finding of sellar enlargement, growth of the area of the skull that contains the pituitary gland. The major event in the timeline of scientific research was Pierre Marie's creation of the diagnostic term "acromegaly" in 1886 [3]. This marked the first time that the characteristics and symptoms of the condition were succinctly summarized and published, although works before Marie's had mentioned many of the same symptoms in patients displaying gigantism [3]. In the years after Marie's paper, investigators began to understand that tumors of the pituitary caused glandular enlargement and were the root of the disease, dispelling previously held notions that they were simply by-products of gigantism. The debate still raged about the relationship between acromegaly and gigantism. At first, Marie believed acromegaly to be pathological, while gigantism was simply an extreme of normal human development. It became apparent after inspecting famous giants' skeletons that the disorders had a "pathogenetic mechanism, but differed with regard to the age of onset." The consensus

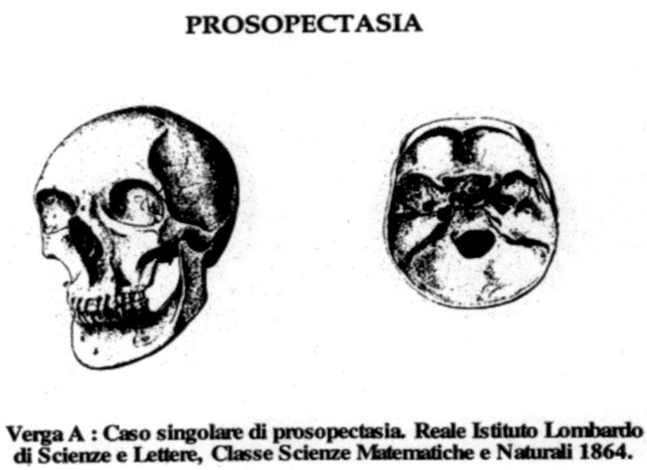

Figure 1. Verga's description of prosopectasia (Author's collection).

was that gigantism has an earlier onset than acromegaly, appearing while the individual is still growing, but that acromegaly occurs after puberty when the person had completed normal growth [3].

The first decade of the 1900s brought concentrated emphasis on the underlying pathological causes behind acromegaly, expanding on the identification of the pituitary as the affected area. This research became part of the basis for the entire "hormone theory." In 1902, E.H. Starling and W.M. Bayliss conducted an experiment in which they injected duodenal extract into a dog intestine, causing the pancreas to become activated and to secrete what was later termed "secretin." [4] Three years later, with the advice of William Hardy, Starling became the first to use the term "hormone" to describe this phenomenon "in which substances produced at one site had the ability to bring about physiological changes at a distant site without a direct neural stimulus." [4] At this point, four major theories of the pituitary's relationship to gigantism and acromegaly had emerged. The first, most notably supported by Marie himself, was that pituitary hyposecretion was the cause. Rebuking this notion, distinguished members of the field, including Massalongo, Tamburini, Benda, Modena, and Fisher, believed that acromegaly was due to pituitary hypersecretion [4]. A third theory, supported by Gauthier, Strumpell, Vassale, and Guerrini, was that it was merely the result of a nutritional disorder and that oversized pituitary fossae were by-products of the disease. Finally, a fourth camp maintained that there was no causation whatsoever between the pituitary and acromegaly.

No one was more influential with his or her work on the pituitary than Dr. Harvey Cushing, author of *The Pituitary Body and Its Disorders*, published in 1912 [4]. Cushing was a proponent of the second theory that an overactive pituitary led to acromegaly and gigantism. The detail in his case studies was second to none, and with his meticulous research, he was able to compile a comprehensive analysis of the disease's true nature. In fact, Cushing became the first person to open the skull of the original Irish Giant, Charles Byrne, in 1909, over a century after Byrne's death. Still held in Hunter's collection, Byrne's worst fears became a reality when Cushing examined his skull to find that he had, as many had long since assumed, an unnaturally large pituitary fossa. In addition to this momentous discovery, Cushing also described a large number of acromegalic patients in his 1912 book (**Figure 2**).

With the image above, Cushing detailed one of the more striking aspects of the disease, the physiological changes to which the affected body is subjected. This instance in particular, which was the first to be mentioned in his long list of case studies, shows a man who would have been described as simply a "normal giant" before the onset of the disease [5]. By this, Cushing meant that while he was an outlier in terms of height before he was afflicted, and this was due to natural growth that did not have anything to do with an enlargement of the pituitary. It was also at this time that, building upon Starling and Bayliss's work on hormones, Cushing became the first to posit that the pituitary was responsible for secreting a "hormone of growth," a massive step toward what would prove to be the correct understanding of gigantism and acromegaly. The way in which modern medicine understands and treats acromegaly and gigantism would not have been possible without each person, professional, and patient, mentioned in this book, as well as countless others who go unmentioned, who are all owed a great deal of gratitude for their contributions.

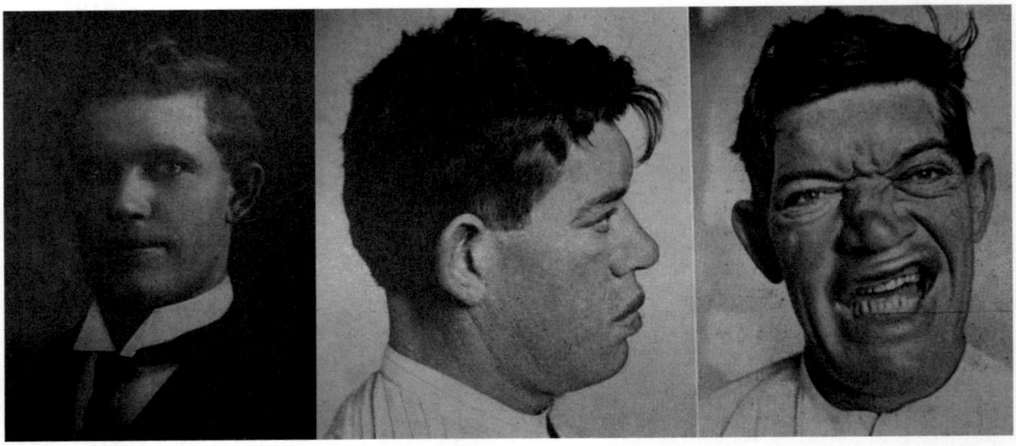

Figure 2. One of Cushing's acromegaly patients from 1910, "M. Van W.," the picture on the left shows the subject pre-acromegaly at age 25. The middle and right pictures show the same man just 10 years later at 35, with obvious acromegalic changes [4].

2. Making the diagnosis

For most patients, acromegaly is a subtle and slowly progressive illness. The clinical findings evolve so slowly that it is often 5–10 years or more before patients seek medical attention. The primary symptoms and signs of acromegaly are listed in **Table 1**. They include progressive enlargement of facial features, hands, and feet; enlargement of the jaw with spacing of the teeth and malocclusion of bite; increased perspiration, with oily skin and a tendency to have acne and skin tags; joint pains; low-back pain; and headache [6].

There are a number of comorbidities characteristic of acromegaly [7]. They include elevated blood pressure, diabetes mellitus, obstructive sleep apnea (OSA), snoring, enlargement of the tongue and upper airway structures, hyperlipidemia, and, in some cases, cardiomyopathy. They are listed in **Table 2**.

A variety of laboratory testing abnormalities can occur in patients with acromegaly. The cardinal features are elevation of serum growth hormone (GH) and IGF-1. Elevations in these hormones are present in patients with active acromegaly, and they are essential for making the diagnosis. Some patients may have elevations in prolactin as well. Pressure on the normal pituitary gland from the tumor can produce a decrease in cortisol, thyroid hormones, and testosterone levels, and abnormalities of gonadotropin hormones can produce fertility problems in women.

Because the location of the pituitary tumor that produces acromegaly is at the base of the skull in the area called the sella turcica, imaging diagnosis is routinely done by magnetic resonance imaging (MRI). Occasionally other imaging studies are helpful in making the diagnosis and in planning treatment. These include computerized tomography (CT) scans to accurately evaluate bony structures, angiography to delineate the vascular elements around the area of the tumor, and rarely nuclear imaging studies such as PET scans [7, 8]. A typical pituitary tumor (macroadenoma) producing acromegaly is seen in **Figure 3**.

Excessive growth: height, hands, feet, hat size, facial features (brow, nose, lips, tongue, jaw), joints (arthropathies), acral bones
Oily skin, acne, excessive sweating (hyperhidrosis), skin tags
Dental gapping, malocclusion
Headache, chest pain
Carpal tunnel syndrome

Table 1. Symptoms and signs of acromegaly.

Hypertension, cardiomyopathy
Diabetes mellitus
Obstructive sleep apnea
Hyperlipidemia
Visual loss (from tumor growth)
Colonic polyps

Table 2. Comorbidities of acromegaly.

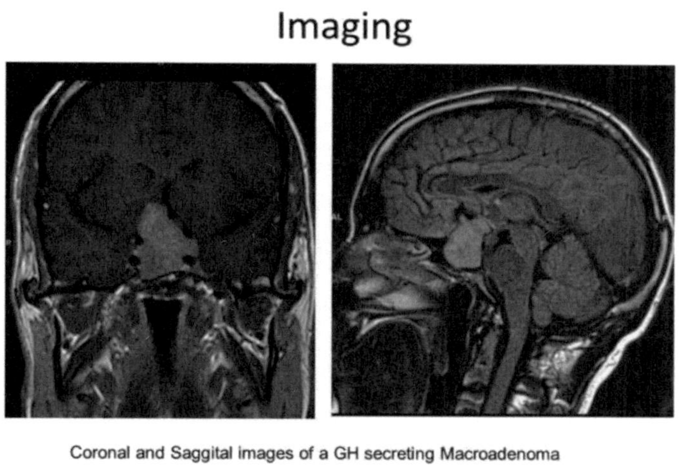

Figure 3. MRI images of a large invasive GH macroadenoma.

3. Classification of growth hormone-secreting tumors in acromegaly

There are two basic characterizations of the size of pituitary tumors. Microadenomas are tumors that are less than 10 mm in maximum diameter. Macroadenomas are those tumors 10 mm or more in maximum diameter. There is also a characterization of uncommon "giant" adenomas that are defined as being 3 or 4 cm in maximum diameter. A further classification is related to tumor cell invasion of the structures around the pituitary. These include invasion of the dural membranes surrounding the pituitary and invasion of the cavernous sinuses on either side of the pituitary (Knosp grading) [9]. Tumors that extend above the pituitary into the suprasellar space can come in contact with the optic chiasm and produce progressive visual loss. The size and stage of these tumors help determine both the goals of surgery and the outcomes for the patients. Occasionally, a pituitary tumor may develop what is called pituitary tumor apoplexy [10] wherein there is hemorrhage into the tumor with rapid enlargement, sometimes involving an emergency situation requiring prompt surgery and prompt cortisol replacement.

4. Indications for surgical management

For the majority of patients, the presence of active acromegaly alone is the indication for surgery, in those patients well enough to undergo anesthesia and the surgical procedure. In addition to halting the relentless progress of acromegaly, successful surgical removal is considered to be "first-line" management [11] and often can also correct visual loss and ameliorate intractable and life-threatening comorbidities. Adjunctive and second-line therapies include various forms of radiation therapy and a number of pharmacologic approaches that are helpful when surgery is either contraindicated or becomes ineffective. Ultimately, the goal is improving the quality of life of our patients with acromegaly.

5. Preoperative evaluation and preparation

In patients being considered for general anesthesia and surgery, a careful preoperative evaluation must be performed [12, 13]. This includes obtaining a full panel of pituitary-focused laboratory testing, with repletion of any hormones that may be deficient, particularly cortisol and thyroid hormone. Repletion of thyroid deficiency must be handled very slowly, as the associated increase in metabolic rate may require adding supplementary cortisol to cover the stress of surgery. It is also important to note that the serum chemistries are in the normal range, especially sodium, potassium, and calcium.

Patients with significant hypertension need to be controlled, and those with a risk of cardiomyopathy must be fully evaluated by a cardiologist. Those patients with diabetes mellitus will need to be managed throughout the surgery and hospitalization to maintain satisfactory glucose levels. Patients with symptomatic obstructive sleep apnea may require particular attention with regard to airway management during surgery and in the postoperative period. It is desirable to alert the anesthesia team in advance for patients who have acromegaly. Acromegaly patients often have difficult airways and may require awake fiber-optic intubation. If the imaging studies show that there is a more than the usual risk of damage to blood vessels in the region of the pituitary, particularly the carotid arteries, an arterial line may be a useful adjunct during anesthesia and postoperatively when and if intensive care unit observation might be necessary. Management of intraoperative fluids and postoperative intake and output of fluids is a critical part of the recovery process for the patients, many of whom will require a urinary catheter during the operative and the postoperative periods.

In some cases of large, invasive, suprasellar GH-secreting tumors, preoperative medical therapy can be useful in shrinking the size of the tumor, making it smaller and safer to remove surgically (**Figure 4**).

The patient is a 32-year-old aviator. After the onset of loss of libido 8 years prior to surgery, he noted the progressive onset of evolving symptoms, including increased shoe and hat size,

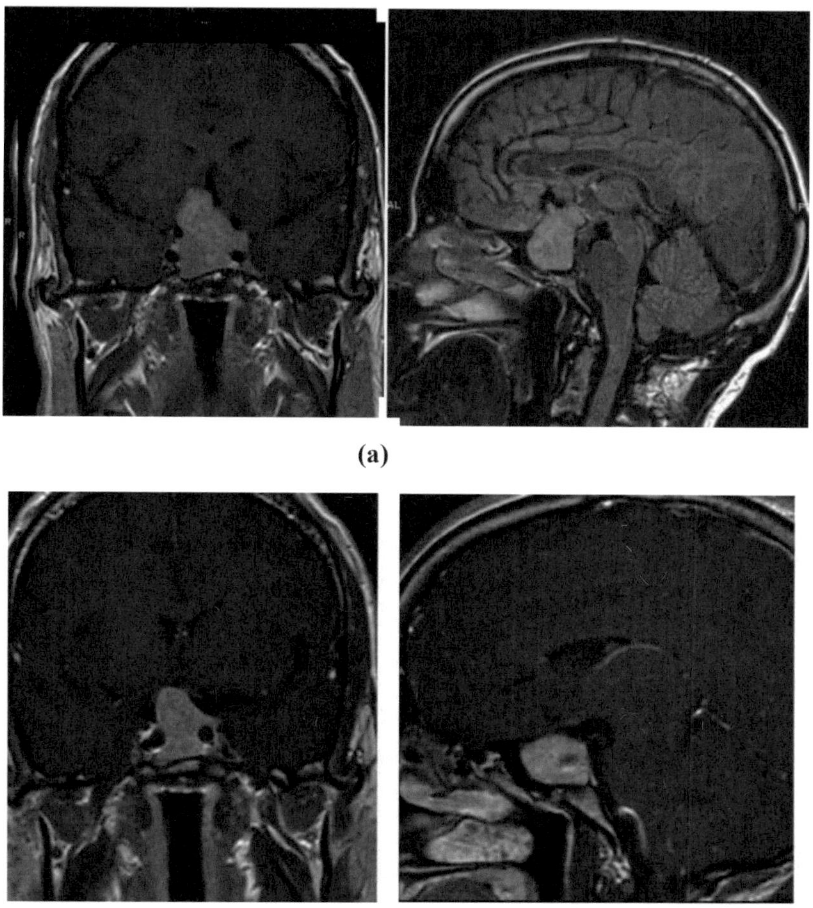

(a)

(b)

Figure 4. Case illustration. (a) Pre-treatment coronal and sagittal images of invasive GH macroadenoma as seen in **Figure 3**. (b) Post-treatment coronal and sagittal images after 3 months of Lanreotide producing major shrinkage, facilitating the subsequent operation (See Section 9). Postoperatively he had normalization of Growth Hormone and IGF-1, and is back flying airplanes!

jaw enlargement, frontal bossing, skin tags, decreased muscle mass, hyperhidrosis, and loss of energy and increasing fatigue. Visual examination revealed 20/20 acuity, bitemporal visual field loss, and decreased retinal fiber layer on ocular computerized tomography. Laboratory investigation revealed low testosterone, FSH, and LH, slightly elevated prolactin at 21.3, low cortisol at 3.6, and elevated growth hormone and IGF-1 at 3.3 and 632, respectively. After 3 months of treatment with lanreotide (Somatostatin analog), the tumor decreased in size and became more amenable to thorough surgical removal.

6. Surgery: methods and considerations

There are two basic routes of access for surgery on patients with acromegaly. Currently, the most utilized is a transnasal transsphenoidal approach using either the operating endoscope or the operating microscope for visualization [8, 14]. Large tumors that extend into the intracranial space and involve the brain, optic chiasm, and major blood vessels are often treated with a craniotomy, so that intracranial structures in danger can be fully visualized in a safe fashion. Because the access to the pituitary is through the nose and the sphenoid sinus, it is often helpful to have the assistance of a qualified otorhinolaryngologist to assist with problems such as nasal septal deviations, septal spurs, imperfect pneumatization of the sphenoid sinus, and other obstacles that may appear during the approach [15]. Patients with acromegaly often have unusually stout bony structures and robust nasal and sinus mucosa which can account for significant bleeding if not carefully controlled. Once the sella turcica has been opened, the dura of the pituitary is incised, and the pituitary tumor is encountered. Every effort is made to spare normal pituitary gland and to accomplish a thorough removal of the growth hormone-secreting pituitary adenoma. Occasionally the tumors are invasive of the dura and adjacent structures. Removal of these portions can increase the risks of surgery but may be essential for developing a complete remission of acromegaly. Some tumors perforate the diaphragm of the sella and after their removal can result in an intraoperative spinal fluid leak. These leaks must be controlled to avoid meningitis. A practical method is to utilize fat taken from the abdomen to fill the empty space left by removing the tumor and secure this leak in an effective fashion [8]. The area of leakage through the sella can also be reinforced with a carefully constructed nasal septal flap [15]. This strategy for repair has been highly effective in preventing postoperative spinal fluid leakage and meningitis. The duration of surgery is usually less than 3 hours, and patients awaken promptly after recovering from anesthesia.

7. Pathology of pituitary tumors in acromegaly

Tumor specimens from surgery are analyzed with great care. Using immunocytochemical techniques, most of the tumors can be fully characterized [16]. The majority express growth hormone only. Because the tumors that produce acromegaly and elevated prolactin secretion come from the same cell line, a number of them are characterized as growth hormone-prolactin staining where some of the tumor cells will stain for one and/or the other of those two hormones. Another less common variant is the mammosomatotroph tumor where each tumor cell can express both growth hormone and prolactin. There is also an acidophil stem cell tumor that is a primitive variant of the latter. The hormone staining is related to the granules within the tumor cell cytoplasm, and they can be classified as either densely granulated or sparsely granulated, with some evidence that the sparsely granulated tumor cells are more aggressive. These tumors producing acromegaly, including the plurihormonal variant, are derived from a cell lineage expressing the Pit-1 transcription promoter. Additionally, the mitotic index is evaluated and the proliferation index of the tumor cells is characterized by MIB-1 staining. These studies are very helpful in correlation with the clinical course of the patients postoperatively.

8. Potential risks and complications of surgery

In experienced hands, the potential risk of serious complications and adverse events is less than 2%. There are, however, potential problems that must be considered and measures taken for prevention of complications [8].

There is a risk of infection, including meningitis, and this may be associated with a spinal fluid leak that ultimately will need repair. Vascular complications can occur and include injury to the carotid arteries, other sources of bleeding from peripheral arteries, veins, and mucous membranes. These can result in vasospasm, stroke, and postoperative epistaxis. Problems with fluid balance can occur, particularly if the posterior pituitary gland or the infundibulum is injured during the operation. This can result in diabetes insipidus which must be carefully treated until it resolves or is corrected by medication with DDAVP. Another issue with regard to fluid balance is the syndrome of inappropriate secretion of ADH (SIADH) which can result in symptomatic hyponatremia which must be carefully and slowly corrected in order to avoid serious problems [17].

9. Medical management of acromegaly

Careful studies of the biology and pathology of growth hormone-secreting pituitary tumors in acromegaly have led to a number of medical strategies for assisting in the treatment of this disorder [5, 11, 13, 18]. The tumor cells that produce increased amounts of growth hormone and prolactin are derived from the same cell lineage. For that reason, a dopamine agonist which is used to treat hyperprolactinemia is moderately effective in helping to control acromegaly. The most commonly used dopamine agonist preparation is cabergoline, usually given by mouth twice a week, and it is usually well-tolerated. Another class of medical agents consists of somatostatin analogs such as octreotide or lanreotide [5]. They have greater effectiveness than cabergoline and also have the possibility of shrinking the size of some growth hormone-secreting pituitary tumors. They are effective in approximately 60% of patients. Another class of drug to treat acromegaly is pegvisomant [18], a growth hormone receptor antagonist. It is given by injection, usually on a daily basis, and is exceedingly expensive at this time. It can be used in combination with somatostatin analogs, improving on the individual results of the two drugs. None of these medical therapies is completely free of side effects.

10. Adjunctive radiation therapy

Another second-line therapy is the use of radiation, which can be delivered in a variety of different timing schedules and with variations in the radiation physics in a number of different modalities that are currently in use [19, 20]. Conventional fractionated teletherapy has been used for some time but currently is being supplanted by more focused methodologies termed stereotactic radiosurgery. The radiosurgical methods include the Gamma Knife, CyberKnife, linear accelerator with multileaf collimator, the proton beam, and the carbon ion beam. Some of these can be given by "single shots" or by fractionation. Each of the modalities has its advantages and disadvantages. With modern techniques, the risks of damage to surrounding neural structures, including the optic nerves and chiasm, and delayed appearance of radiation-induced neoplasms are quite low. In patients with acromegaly, there is a fairly long delay time for the radiation to gradually lower the growth hormone and IGF-1. Most of the techniques currently utilized are effective but are also associated with a significant degree of radiation-induced hypopituitarism regarding the other hormones.

11. Criteria for remission after therapy

Clinical signs of remission of acromegaly tend to occur fairly early in those patients who have a satisfactory result of treatment. Some clinical signs improve rapidly, especially difficulty with the upper airway and snoring, along with the diminishment of excessive perspiration, and gradual improvements in the soft tissue issues affecting the hands, feet, and facial features. Headache is often alleviated. Arthropathies tend to linger much longer, but ultimately improve in many patients. Some patients with hypertension and diabetes will manifest progressive clinical improvement, which gradually occurs over time. More than 80% of patients who have visual compromise are improved postoperatively.

Biochemical remission is critical, and normalization of the serum levels of growth hormone and IGF-1 is monitored to assess the pace and degree of remission [11, 14, 15]. It often takes 3 months or more for IGF-1 to reach its nadir after surgery, but the growth hormone response occurs more promptly. Additionally, the dynamics of growth hormone regulation can be measured by performing an oral glucose tolerance test and measuring the response of growth hormone, which should become significantly decreased after a glucose challenge.

Ordinarily, we wait 3 months to obtain a definitive postoperative MRI scan which will serve as a baseline for the future. For the initial few years, annual MRI studies are often recommended, and they are done if there is not a complete remission or if there is a recurrence of

http://dx.doi.org/10.5772/intechopen.91430

symptoms and/or abnormal laboratory results. We recommend that the pituitary hormones and IGF-1 be measured every 6 months for the first several years.

12. Outcomes of surgical management of acromegaly

Initial remission of acromegaly as measured by clinical and biochemical criteria occurs in 50–60% of macroadenomas and 80–90% of microadenomas [11, 13, 21]. Results are less effective when the surgeon is dealing with large macroadenomas or tumors that are invasive of surrounding structures. Postoperative improvement in the management of diabetes mellitus and hypertension is seen in approximately 75% of patients. The majority of patients who present with obstructive sleep apnea develop improvement after successful surgery. Although pituitary adenomas are generally benign tumors that do not progress to malignancy, tumor recurrence does develop in some patients over time. After initial successful surgery, recurrence will develop in approximately 8% of patients within the first 10 years following successful surgery. Because the objective of all forms of management of acromegaly are to improve the quality of life of the patient, a number of questionnaires and instruments have been developed [21, 22] to measure quality of life, and they provide good insight as to the results of current therapy and for areas with needs for improvement. Studies have demonstrated that sustained remission of patients with acromegaly provides mortality figures similar to the general age-matched population [23]. There is evidence to suggest that significant surgical experience is a major factor in achieving optimal outcomes [23]. Although great strides have occurred, continuous development of knowledge concerning the genetics and molecular biology of acromegaly will undoubtedly provide us with more versatile and effective avenues of progress.

13. Conclusion

Acromegaly is the current quintessential example of a hyperfunctioning tumor of the pituitary gland. It is usually a benign tumor; however, it has multiple side effects and comorbidities that threaten the life and wellbeing of the patient. Steady progress has been made since its original description in understanding the pathophysiology of pituitary adenomas. We have learned a great deal about the molecular biology and hypothalamic regulation of pituitary cells that secrete growth hormone and induce elevations in IGF-1. At present, the first-line therapy is surgery to remove the tumor, usually by the endonasal transsphenoidal approach, often with the aid of a surgical endoscope. The results of surgical management are generally excellent, and techniques and outcomes are steadily improving. Initial criteria for the development of centers of excellence for pituitary adenoma diagnosis and treatment are being developed [24]. Surely, further scientific investigation will improve the nonsurgical adjunctive management of growth hormone-secreting pituitary tumors, primarily using appropriate drugs that target the physiological and genetic mechanisms of these tumors that secrete excess growth hormone.

Author details

John L. Kilgallon[1] and Edward R. Laws[2*]

*Address all correspondence to: elaws@bwh.harvard.edu

1 Princeton University, New Jersey, USA

2 Harvard Medical School, Boston, Massachusetts, USA

References

[1] Muinzer TL. A grave situation: An examination of the legal issues raised by the life and death of Charles Byrne, the 'Irish Giant'. International Journal of Cultural Property. 2013;**20**(1):26

[2] Mammis A, Eloy JA, Liu JK. Early descriptions of acromegaly and gigantism and their historical evolution as clinical entities. Neurosurgical Focus. 2010;**29**(4):1

[3] Herder WW. Acromegaly and gigantism in the medical literature. Case descriptions in the era before and the early years after the initial publication of Pierre Marie (1886). Pituitary. 2009;**12**(3):236

[4] Cushing H. The Pituitary Body and Its Disorders. London: J.B. Lippincott; 1912. p. 30

[5] Colao A, Grasso L, Giustina Q, Melmed S, Chanson P, Pereira A, et al. Acromegaly. Nature Reviews Disease Primers. 2019;**5**:20

[6] Iuliano SI, Laws ER. Recognizing the clinical manifestations of acromegaly: Case studies. Journal of the American Association of Nurse Practitioners. 2013;**26**(3):136

[7] Powlson AS, Gurnell M. Cardiovascular disease and sleep-disordered breathing in acromegaly. Neuroendocrinology. 2016;**103**:75-85

[8] Laws ER Jr, Cote DJ, Iuliano S. Transsphenoidal surgery for acromegaly. In: Laws ER Jr, editor. Transsphenoidal Surgery. New York: Springer International; 2017. DOI: 10.1007/978-3-319-56691-7_25

[9] Knosp E, Steiner E, Kitz K, Matula C. Pituitary adenomas with invasion of the cavernous sinus space: A magnetic resonance imaging classification compared with surgical findings. Neurosurgery. 1993;**33**:610-617

[10] Semple PL, Jane JA Jr, Lopes MB, Laws ER. Pituitary apoplexy: Correlation between magnetic resonance imaging and histopathological results. Journal of Neurosurgery. 2008;**108**:909-915

[11] Katznelson L, Laws ER, Melmed S, Molitch ME, Murad MH, Utz A, et al. Acromegaly: An endocrine society clinical practice guideline. The Journal of Clinical Endocrinology and Metabolism. 2014;**99**(11):3933-3951

[12] Melmed S, Colao A, Barkan A, Molitch M, Grossman AB, Kleinberg D, et al. Acromegaly Consensus Group. Guidelines for acromegaly management: An update. The Journal of Clinical Endocrinology and Metabolism. 2009;**94**:1509-1517

[13] Nachtigall L, Delgado A, Swearingen B, Lee H, Zerikly R, Klibanski A. Extensive clinical experience: Changing patterns in diagnosis and therapy of acromegaly over two decades. The Journal of Clinical Endocrinology and Metabolism. 2008;**93**:2035-2041

[14] Kreutzer J, Vance M, Lopes M, Laws ER Jr. Surgical management of GH-secreting pituitary adenomas: An outcome study using modern remission criteria. The Journal of Clinical Endocrinology and Metabolism. 2001;**86**:4072-4077

[15] Jane JA, Starke RM, Elzoghby MA, Reames DL, Payne SC, Thorner MO, et al. Endoscopic transsphenoidal surgery for acromegaly: Remission using modern criteria, complications, and predictors of outcome. The Journal of Clinical Endocrinology and Metabolism. 2011;**96**(9):2732-2740

[16] Zada G, Cavallo LM, Esposito F, Fernandez-Jimenez JC, Tasiou A, De Angelis M, et al. Endoscopic transsphenoidal surgery in patients with longstanding acromegaly: Operative strategies for overcoming technically challenging anatomical variations. Neurosurgical Focus. 2010;**29**(4)

[17] Laws ER, Lopes MB. The new WHO classification of pituitary adenomas: Highlights and areas of controversy. Acta Neuropathologica. 2006;**111**:80-81

[18] Buchfelder M, van der Lely AJ, Biller B, et al. Long-term treatment with pegvisomant: From observations from 2090 patients in ACROSTUDY. European Journal of Endocrinology. 2018;**179**:419-427

[19] Ding D, Mehta GU, Patibandla MR, et al. Stereotactic radiosurgery for acromegaly: An international multicenter retrospective cohort study. Neurosurgery. 2019;**84**:717-725

[20] Jagnnathan J, Sheehan JP, Pouratian N, Laws ER, Steiner L, Vance ML. Gamma knife radiosurgery for acromegaly: Outcomes after failed transsphenoidal surgery. Neurosurgery. 2008;**62**(6):1262-1269

[21] van der Lely A, Gomez R, Pleil A, et al. Development of ACRODAT, a new software medical device to assess disease activity in patients with acromegaly. Pituitary. 2017;**20**(22): 692-701

[22] Giustina A, Bronstein M, et al. Staging and managing patients with acromegaly in clinical practice: Baseline data from the SAGIT validation study. Pituitary. 2019;**22**:476-487

[23] Swearingen B, Barker F, Katznelson L, Biller B, Grinspoon S, Klibanski A, et al. Long term mortality after transsphenoidal surgery and adjunctive therapy for acromegaly. The Journal of Clinical Endocrinology and Metabolism. 1998;**83**:3419-3426

[24] Casaneuva F, Barkan A, Buchfelder M, et al. Criteria for the definition of pituitary tumor centers of excellence (PTCOE): A pituitary society statement. Pituitary. 2017: 489-498